THE
SKINNY
JEANS
DIET

THE SKINNY JEANS DIET

Change Your Thinking,
Change Your Eating,
and **FINALLY**
Fit into Your Pants!

Lyssa Weiss, M.S., R.D., C.D.N.

wm

WILLIAM MORROW
An Imprint of HarperCollins*Publishers*

This book is written as a source of information only. The information contained in this book should by no means be considered a substitute for the advice of a qualified medical professional, who should always be consulted before beginning any new diet, exercise, or other health program.

All efforts have been made to ensure the accuracy of the information contained in this book as of the date published. The author and the publisher expressly disclaim responsibility for any adverse effects arising from the use or application of the information contained herein.

THE SKINNY JEANS DIET. Copyright © 2014 by Lyssa Weiss. All rights reserved. Printed in the United States of America. No part of this book may be used or reproduced in any manner whatsoever without written permission except in the case of brief quotations embodied in critical articles and reviews. For information address HarperCollins Publishers, 195 Broadway, New York, NY 10007.

HarperCollins books may be purchased for educational, business, or sales promotional use. For information please e-mail the Special Markets Department at SPsales@harpercollins.com.

FIRST EDITION

Designed by Diahann Sturge

Illustration © Pixel Embargo/Shutterstock, Inc.

Library of Congress Cataloging-in-Publication Data has been applied for.

ISBN 978-0-06-213560-5

14 15 16 17 18   OV/RRD   10 9 8 7 6 5 4 3 2 1

To my husband, Stephen; my beautiful children,
Alix and Evan; and my extraordinary parents,
Gari and Ira Dansky. I love you all so much.
You take my breath away.

Contents

Contents

THE
SKINNY
JEANS
DIET

Introduction

- Do you obsess about brownies? Do chocolate chip cookies drive you to distraction?
- Have you ever tried to get "in the mood" and realized that the only thing you were in the mood for was a bag of potato chips?
- Have you ever finished a slice of half-eaten cake from the trash or dipped into your kids' Halloween stash? Do you binge on batter, chow down on Cheetos, or munch mercilessly on M&Ms?
- Do you have a favorite dress that now barely fits over your arm, let alone your thighs?
- Do your jeans let out a sigh of relief after you take them off?

If you answered yes to one or more of these questions, then you need to get clear on one thing: you've got a problem with food. But it doesn't have to be that way. *Food doesn't have to rule your life. Finally, you can learn to rule food.*

The Skinny Jeans Diet is a back-to-basics, "how much can I eat and still fit into my pants" survival guide for the millions of women who struggle every day with their weight. In the pages of this book, you'll discover essential tips, tricks, eating strategies, and recipes that have helped hundreds of women lose and, more important, keep off thousands of pounds. This is the first and only eating plan that's built not around some arbitrary, government-structured pyramid or "food plate," but around you. The Skinny Jeans Diet teaches you how to live thin . . . forever. And along the way, you'll learn how to fit back into your skinny jeans. What could be better than that?

Food is our best friend and also our worst enemy. In fact, it may be our most complicated and troubled relationship. From childhood, we're taught that food isn't just food. It's a reward after a tough day, a treat for a job well done, and a pick-me-up when we're down. It's love, support, and comfort.

However, if you think of food as a source of love, I have news for you: it's not. Food, as I tell my clients, is the ultimate booby prize. For millions of dieters, it's a source of self-loathing, poor body image, lack of self-esteem, and ill health. The Skinny Jeans Diet is for any woman who wants to break free of a destructive and demoralizing relationship with food. It's self-empowerment for ending the dangerous and disheartening cycle of losing and regaining weight. The Skinny Jeans Diet gives you the keys to the kingdom—the essential knowledge you need to live comfortably in a world in which food temptation lurks around every corner.

But the Skinny Jeans Diet isn't just an eating plan. Anyone can tell you what to eat. Scour the Internet, browse the aisles of your local bookstore, visit a nutritionist, watch the morning talk shows, pick up a women's magazine—you'll find more than enough sound, reliable information about what and what not to eat to lose weight. Creating a diet for my clients is the easy part. *Getting them to stick to a diet is a whole other matter!*

That's why the Skinny Jeans Diet is, at its core, a *thinking plan.* I guarantee that if you don't change your fundamental thoughts, feelings, and assumptions about food, then you'll end up just another failed dieter. And you'll have millions to keep you company.

Crazy Girl Gone Good

WHEN IT COMES TO DIETING, I'VE DONE IT ALL. I'VE LOST AND gained weight more times than Lady Gaga has changed outfits. I've been really fat, and I've been super-skinny. I've been bulimic, and I've been anorexic. I binged and I purged. I shrank to a size 2 and ballooned to a size 14. I've counted points, eaten like a cavewoman, dined at South Beach, lived on cabbage soup, eaten for my blood type, and been in the Zone. In my darkest moments, I'm still a weight-crazed, food-obsessed lunatic. In other words, *I'm just like you!* Here is just a smattering of my food "crimes":

- Picking the chocolate coating off of a dozen or so ice cream bars
- Licking the vanilla glaze off of an entire box of Munchkins . . . and then polishing it off with a sugar cube
- Buying two batches of cookie mix . . . and putting just one in the oven (can you guess where the other batch went?)

My obsession with food started early. By the time I reached the sixth grade, my rapidly developing body had become a source of shame and embarrassment, causing me to stand out from the other girls. Needless to say, I felt intensely self-conscious. From tight bras and big shirts to slouching and wearing loose-fitting pants, I did everything imaginable to hide my shape.

This was when I also discovered that food was an ideal escape. It never talked back, didn't put me down, didn't break my heart, and provided immediate relief from whatever unpleasant feeling or experience I was dealing with. Whenever I felt self-conscious, uncomfortable, stressed out, or anxious, I'd eat. Food became the perfect outlet for my inner turmoil. Even fantasies of fitting into a pretty dress couldn't pry me away from a box of doughnuts or a package of Pillsbury cookie dough. And though all of my binges were always followed by shame, guilt, self-loathing, and social isolation, I just couldn't seem to stop myself.

As I got older my eating caused me to stand out—because I couldn't wear what was cool. When tight-fitting, acid-washed jeans were all the rage, I wore flares. To balance out my heavy frame, I wore shoulder pads . . . long after everyone else had put 1980s style in the rearview mirror.

There isn't a diet program I haven't tried, weight loss support group I haven't attended, or "lite" food I haven't sampled—all resulting in failure. At breakfast I'd dream about lunch, at lunch I'd fantasize about dinner, and at dinner I'd already be thinking about what I could eat during my regular late-night refrigerator raids. I'd dream up occasions that called for cookies—just so I could binge on raw batter. I stashed bags of chips under my bed. I strategically placed candy all over the house and then hid the wrappers in my pillowcase to hide my shame.

Of course, none of this worked. I hated myself and hated the way I looked. My confidence plummeted, and my self-esteem was nonexistent. My life was like a runaway train.

How did I stop?

By learning a better way. I became a nutritionist. When I started my nutrition studies, it was clear that I'd been preparing to be a nutritionist my whole life. After living through what seemed like a lifetime's worth of eating disorders and experiencing my own issues with food, I soon realized my calling.

Nutrition wasn't just something I wanted to do—it was something I needed to do. Unlike many of my colleagues who entered the field to help others—to spread the gospel of healthy nutrition—I had goals early on that weren't nearly as lofty. I became a nutritionist in large part to heal myself.

The idea that what we put in our mouths plays a critical role in our overall well-being was something I always was tangentially aware of, but couldn't do anything about because I had spent the better part of my life mired in "fat thinking." It became obvious that I had never developed a healthy relationship with food, no matter how much weight I lost.

To heal myself I had to go beyond the scale. I was torturing myself with food because I was living with the belief that no matter how hard I tried, I would never measure up. The idea that I should be different from who I am created a void, which I unhappily filled with food. The yo-yo cycle of losing and regaining weight had less to do with cookies and potato chips and more to do with how I saw myself and my place in the world. I was doing everything possible to control my external environment because my internal world was careening out of control.

Someone a lot wiser than me once said that we define ourselves in large measure by how we respond to the world around us. No one is immune to adversity. As Carl Jung stated, "Nobody, as long as he moves about among the chaotic currents of life, is without trouble." The number of negative things that can happen to us in just a single day seems endless. Often, you can't control what happens to you. However, you can almost always control how you react. For me, it took many years of sadness and frustration to learn this valuable lesson. To master my relationship with food I first had to master my relationship with myself. Self-mastery, I would soon discover, is the key to happiness in this life. As the great Taoist sage Lao Tzu observed, "He who controls others may be powerful, but he who has mastered himself is mightier still."

After I started graduate school, something amazing happened. I got smart. For the first time I saw my weight problems for what they were: a disease of thinking. As my head got lighter my body followed suit. Using real-life strategies, cutting-edge nutrition knowledge, and great-tasting light foods and recipes, I finally discovered how to live thin.

You see, even if you lose the weight, you don't lose the problem. Weight isn't the issue for most dieters. It's a symptom—a symptom of being out of control with food. What you put in your mouth is always secondary to what you put in your head.

The Skinny Jeans Mind-set

THE FANCY DIPLOMAS LINING MY OFFICE WALL MAY SAY THAT I'M A nutritionist, but more important to my ability to help you is the fact that I *am* you. I've been where you are. I've journeyed to diet hell and lived to tell the tale. I've won where so many have lost. Now I want to help you do the same. Scales, calorie charts, and measuring tapes aren't the tools of my trade. I use practicality, presence of mind, and a healthy dose of common sense to rule the world of food. This book will show you how I did it and how you too can get thin and *stay that way*.

Today I have a kick-ass closet full of stylish and sexy clothes. I wear the skinniest skinny jeans. Those horrible shoulder pads, too-tight brassieres, and baggy shirts are nowhere in sight—and never again will be part of my wardrobe. Most of all, I'm present in my life—and because of that, I'm content and motivated every day to take care of the gifts I've been given.

I created the Skinny Jeans Diet for anyone who wants to live thin, thrive in the world of food, and fit into her favorite pants. Enjoy the book, and use everything in it to be the healthiest, the happiest, the most gorgeous you imaginable.

PART ONE

Living Skinny

CHAPTER 1

Bad Boyfriends: Your Personal Relationship with Food

The definition of insanity is doing the same thing over and over again and expecting different results.

—Albert Einstein

W E'VE ALL BEEN THERE. HE APPEARS, AS IF BY MAGIC, while you're waiting on an impossibly long line for the day's first double latte. You can't help but stare. Your eyes are motionless, your body frozen at the sight of this modern-day Adonis. He's got the perfect jawline, the oh so sexy, slightly disheveled mane, world-class charisma, to-die-for dimples, piercing, ocean-deep blue eyes, and abs that look like they were chiseled out of marble. You don't even know his name, but already you're hooked. He's hot, and you know it (and so does he).

Then he walks over to you and starts making conversation. Your heart sinks in your chest. You stumble for words. Turns out, you hit it off instantly, even though you barely hear a word he's saying. You feel a whole new level of chemistry with this man. He's slightly naughty but also charming and witty. He even offers to buy your coffee. You're swooning, but you have to tone down your feelings. You're entertaining thoughts of bringing him home to meet your folks. This is the boy you always thought you'd marry.

Here's the problem. After just a few dates, you discover that he's deathly allergic to commitment and responsibility. He's constantly out of cash, and you always seem to be picking up the tab. He treats waitstaff and other service people poorly. After sex, he's out the door faster than the time it takes you to tie your shoes. Your friends and family don't like him; you're forever making excuses for him. In fact, you don't even feel that good about yourself around him. Deep down, you know he's 100 percent wrong for you. But you just can't stay away. The confidence, the indifference, the challenge—not to mention the beautiful, wavy Richard Gere hair and killer abs—keep sucking you back in.

For most of us, certain foods are like bad boyfriends. And whatever the type, we just can't seem to stay away. Cookies, buttery dinner rolls, cupcakes, doughnuts, sugary cereal, ice cream, nuts, popcorn, candy—I think you get the picture. These foods—and many others—are our bad boyfriends. We know they're wrong for us, but try as we might, we can't seem to get them out of our lives. Friends and family warn us about them. Our doctors tell us to stop. But we just can't seem to rein ourselves in. They call to us. In their presence, we lose our minds, not to mention our waistlines. We eat too many of them; we binge uncontrollably when they're presented to us. After we're through, we beat ourselves up mercilessly. Every time we hook up, we get ourselves into trouble. No good ever comes of this relationship.

How do you know if your favorite food is a bad boyfriend?

Bad Boyfriends Come in Cute Packages!

WHEN IT COMES TO BAD BOYFRIENDS, PACKAGING IS EVERYTHING. Putting aside (but just for a moment) the perfect dimples, great smile, and tight tush, the bad boyfriend is usually dressed (or undressed as the case may be) to the nines. Custom-made wardrobe, perfectly tousled locks, fab car, and the hottest shades—bad boyfriends are the complete package. It's part of their appeal. It's how they lure you in, even after you've sworn off men for the 18th time in the last two months.

The foods we love to hate are almost always like this. They come in vivid, brightly colored, and attractive packaging that immediately draws us to them whether we're trawling the supermarket aisles or watching television. They arouse our imagination before they stimulate our appetite. Slickly marketed, they encourage us to buy, consume, and ultimately overeat them. Food manufacturers have to sell us their products this way, as Michael Pollan observes in his groundbreaking book *The Omnivore's Dilemma*:

> Try as we might, the average person can eat only about fifteen hundred pounds of food a year. . . . This leaves food companies like General Mills with two choices. They can figure out how to get people to spend more money for the same amount of food. Or they can get us to eat more food than we need. Which do they choose? Why, both, of course. Consumers will only pay so much for an ear of corn. But they can be convinced to pay a lot more for the same corn if it has been turned into a funny shape, sweetened, and brightly colored. The industry calls this "adding value."

This is why food manufacturers spend billions on advertising. They have to convince us that it adds value to turn potatoes into potato chips, corn into sweet kettle corn, or cereal into cereal bars. However, we all know that the only thing being added with these foods is inches to our waistline, especially if that food is a bad boyfriend, which it often is. When was the last time you saw broccoli or asparagus in a brightly colored package? Have you ever seen someone try to "add value" to squash, beets, or turnips?

Is it any wonder we keep returning to our bad boyfriends? They're con artists. It's in their DNA. You can't keep up a pretense of civility with a rattlesnake. Get too close and you'll get bitten. I have clients who try to reason with their bad boyfriends. I remember one client, the director of marketing for a string of fancy day spas, who thought she could talk herself into having just "a little" chocolate even though she'd been overeating it since she was a child and it was the number-one cause of her lifelong struggle with weight. "For 30 years, you've never been able to control yourself around chocolate," I told her. "What makes you think a little cognitive psychology on a Hershey's bar is going to make any difference?"

You know the saying "If it walks like a duck, swims like a duck, and quacks like a duck, then it probably is a duck"? A cookie is a cookie is a cookie, and you will get yourself into a mess *every time* if it's your bad boyfriend! You can change the packaging, throw in a few peanuts, and even add some fiber (there are cookies like that). But at the end of the day, it'll still be a cookie. And if you've been overeating cookies your whole life, then this is your pattern. Just like the bad boyfriend isn't suddenly going to transform into a mensch, the cookie isn't going to morph into a bag of carrots. You've got to change, because the cookie won't. It's like telling a zebra to stop grazing on grass. Offer a zebra the finest pâté, oysters, and caviar, and it will always opt for the grass. This is what zebras do. They eat grass.

A food that causes you to lose control of your eating is going to do what it's always done and give you the results you've always gotten: extra pounds, extra inches, and a first-class ticket to the plus-sized racks. A food you've always overeaten is a no-win situation. As Dr. Phil always says, "How's that working for you?" If you don't come face to face with the reality of how you behave around certain foods, you will never end the destructive cycle of losing and regaining weight.

PACKAGING TIP

If you must have a bad boyfriend in the house, there are steps you can take to make him less alluring. Remember that bad boyfriends frequently come in brightly colored boxes and bags that draw us in. They're designed to get us to buy and overconsume them. Start by taking the food out of its original package and putting it in a plain, opaque container or a Ziploc bag. The food will instantly become less appealing, and you'll certainly lose interest. Just as a boy—even a cute one—in baggy jeans and an old flannel shirt is a lot less appealing than a stud in Armani, Frosted Flakes without Tony the Tiger becomes as boring as cornflakes. No one wants to be bored on a date. But when it comes to our bad boyfriends, dull is good!

Can You Turn It Down?

ARE YOU STRUGGLING TO BREAK IT OFF? IF IT'S A BAD BOYFRIEND, the answer is almost certainly "yes." Breaking it off with the suave Mr. Chips Ahoy! or that handsome Hershey's Kiss is never easy. They call and you answer without fail—every single time. You open a bag to have "just one," then make quick work of the entire sleeve or half the bag. When in your life have you ever been able to have just one? You realize that the "one" cookie you intended to eat quickly became 15 (and 70 percent of the day's calories).

Still, you keep them in your life anyway. What's that all about? "To thine own self be true," said Shakespeare. It's too bad that you turn into a whole other person around cookies. I know you bought those cookies with the best intentions, which is how the road to hell is paved, if I'm not mistaken. But intentions are no match for a habitual lack of control. Few of us have the strength or willpower to turn down a bad boyfriend. If we did, then we wouldn't be struggling with our weight. That's why ending the bad boyfriend habit takes more than determination. It demands a plan!

Reducing temptation is a great trick for staying in control with bad boyfriend foods. This can involve knocking them out of your life altogether (not because you can't eat them but because they're keeping you out of that hot red bikini) or limiting them to carefully controlled situations.

Like many women, my client Sue has rich chocolate desserts and popcorn for bad boyfriends. Years ago, Sue made the very "skinny jeans" decision to swear off popcorn because no matter what tricks she used, she simply couldn't control her consumption of it. On the other hand, Sue feels more in control around chocolate, so instead of forgoing it completely, she allows herself chocolate in carefully controlled circumstances, such as at a party or a restaurant. And when she does opt for chocolate, she limits her choice to lower-calorie alternatives she seldom encounters, like flourless chocolate cake or Jell-O Mousse Temptations—a 60-calorie, single-serving cup of chocolate mousse. Now Sue has her cake and eats it too!

Beauty Is in the Eye of the Beholder

WHEN IT COMES TO OUR PERSONAL RELATIONSHIP WITH FOOD, beauty is truly in the eye of the beholder. A bad boyfriend for one girl may be a keeper for another. I have clients who can stare down a basket of rolls and not give it a second thought, and others who'll demolish an entire loaf of bread in one sitting. If you're still in the dark about which foods cause you to spiral out of control—though most people who take an honest inventory will know which foods those are—ask yourself, *Can I control my eating with this food?* If it's potato chips, that well-intentioned handful of chips may turn into an entire bag, not to mention a week's worth of self-loathing and guilt. Look closely and you'll probably start to see predictable patterns. You may discover that certain foods have always stirred up cravings in you, causing you to overeat. If you find that a single 10-calorie potato chip quickly morphs into a 2,000-calorie monster, then you probably have your answer.

Taking an Honest Inventory

YOU MUST TAKE AN HONEST INVENTORY OF YOUR "BAD BOY-friends" and know that these foods can't (or shouldn't) be a part of your everyday life. If you've had an ongoing, lifelong drama with Peanut M&Ms, for instance, clearly something is amiss.

Looking at the foods that do and don't work for us isn't always easy. This isn't a matter of simply locating the most nutritionally sound foods. Everyone knows an apple is better for your health than a cookie. But many of us eat 20 cookies for every one apple. This is about looking at the foods that do work in your life—and those that don't.

Breaking the Bad Boyfriend Habit

AS WITH A BAD BOYFRIEND, YOUR RELATIONSHIP WITH THESE foods is all out of whack. What do you do?

STEP 1. KNOW WHO YOUR BAD BOYFRIENDS ARE

Weighing protein, tracking points, and counting calories won't do you much good if you don't take a long hard look at which foods work for you and which work against you. This isn't simply about changing your weight or clothing size. Weight is a symptom of a much larger issue. To lose weight and keep it off, you have to change the thinking and behavior that got you into trouble in the first place. And get rid of the idea that you and your ex can just be friends. Your bad boyfriend is a compulsion; otherwise, you would have ditched him the first time he asked to borrow money or cheated on you. By the way, when was the last time you enjoyed just a little of a compulsion?

The first step is to identify *your* bad boyfriends. What are your trigger foods? What are the foods that have always caused you to lose control? Write down some likely suspects and give your list a good hard look. Ask yourself:

- Can you control your eating with this food? Or does "one" quickly turn into an entire sleeve, box, or bag?
- Does this food stir up cravings for more and more? Or worse, does it lead you to other foods? For example, do potato chips stir up interest in other bite-size, crunchy, salty foods, such as pretzels and peanuts? For many of us, crunchy, salty snacks are gateway foods that open the door to other foods that could easily be abused.
- Will this food lead you down the garden path to thin? Or will it push you off the diet wagon after weeks, months, or even years of good behavior?
- Do you often seek out this food when you're stressed, sad, upset, or lonely?
- Is this a food you typically eat alone?
- When you begin a new diet, do you swear off this food, only to find yourself returning to it after you reach your target weight?
- Do you gravitate to this food even if you feel full or you aren't hungry?

If you've answered "yes" to some of these questions about a particular food, it's probably one that's all wrong for you. It goes on your bad boyfriend list.

Step 2. Face What Having a Bad Boyfriend Means

Since the *food* isn't going to change, you must. If you don't come face to face with the reality of how you act around the foods that cause you to lose control, you will *never* reach your ideal weight.

Stop testing yourself to see whether you can handle the risk of being around these foods. You can't and you'll keep failing. Self-sabotage is the undoing of even the most obdurate dieters. If a food is truly a bad boyfriend, then you've got to "wash that man right out of your hair." And leave it out of your shopping cart, and *out* of your house. Don't order it in a restaurant. If your children or spouse come home with one (or more) of your bad boyfriends, get rid of them. If you get a bad boyfriend as a gift, find him a foster home, give him to the mailman, or donate him as a snack for your child's class. And don't make the mistake of saying that you're buying it for someone else.

Remember, however, that it may not be enough to kick your bad boyfriend to the curb or toss him in a garbage pail. He's adept at wooing you. A few minutes of sweet talk and you're going to be asking him for a nightcap. Destroy your bad boyfriend by dumping soap, ketchup, or salt on it—anything to ruin the taste. You may be in agony now, but your scale—and your skinny jeans—will thank you later.

Does breaking the bad boyfriend habit mean that you'll never find true love again? Of course it doesn't. But you will have to be smart about where, when, and how you consume foods on the bad boyfriend list. When it comes to our bad boyfriends, context is everything. There are some girls who have no trouble with a single skinny slice of birthday cake at a party but know better than to keep cake at home, since they'll work a cake down to crumbs in no time flat.

However, with careful planning and an awareness of their personal relationship with food, some girls can have their cake and eat it too, as my client Marni's story demonstrates.

CAN YOU EVER HAVE A BAD BOYFRIEND FOOD?

Marni is a journalist who works from home. She loves her job, but like many writers, Marni sometimes struggles with writer's block. Every time she feels it coming on, she pops into the kitchen for a quick snack. Her writer's block seems to rev up around deadlines. As the pressure increases, so do the number of visits to the kitchen. During one super-stressful week, she plowed through two bags of Twix Mini Bars. Marni convinced herself that her bad boyfriend was helping her get her work done, but all it was doing was distracting her and making her gain weight. Deep down, Marni probably knew her bad boyfriend wasn't doing much good, but in the heat of the moment it made everything easier.

Marni was upset when she came to see me. The first step was to identify the problem—stress eating—and then find more appropriate outlets for her writer's block, such as running errands, taking a walk, or talking on the phone with an old friend, anything to divert her attention away from food.

Second, we discussed keeping the bad boys out of the house altogether and reserving them for special occasions. This could work for Marni, since she abuses chocolate bars only if they're readily available. She'd never run down to the local convenience store for Twix Bars; they have to be lurking nearby. Now Marni no longer keeps candy bars in her home. When her chocolate craving strikes, she buys a single serving of a healthier alternative, such as a protein-rich Questbar Double Chocolate Chunk Protein Bar or a NuGo Slim Brownie Crunch Bar, both of which offer chewy texture and great taste but for a fraction of the calories of traditional chocolate bars. Today Marni, 20 pounds lighter and two dress sizes lower, still keeps company with her bad boyfriend food, but now she's dictating the terms.

STEP 3. DON'T MAKE EXCUSES

Most of us have been socialized to treat food as a reward or a treat. "But it looks so good," we say. Or, "It's a special occasion," "I had a bad day," "It's for the kids," or "I cooked it." Food shouldn't be seen as comfort after a fight with your spouse or a reward after a long week at work. This approach leads to failure.

STEP 4. IT'S NOT JUST ABOUT THE FOOD

Sometimes it's not *what* you eat but *how* you eat that makes all the difference. Your eating preference or style also reveals your bad boyfriend's true colors. I have an older client, Joyce, whose bad boyfriend isn't a particular food but portion control and what I refer to as a "Depression-era food mentality." She told me that she couldn't remember a time when she didn't finish everything on her plate. "I hate throwing food away. It drives me nuts and makes me feel like I'm flushing money down the toilet," said Joyce during our first session.

In truth, Joyce had been "flushing" a lot more down the toilet: doctors' bills, fad diets, therapists' appointments, and exercise equipment were all consequences of not "wasting" food. Today Joyce buys only single-serving portions of her favorite foods, which is a great trick to help anyone avoid overconsumption. After all, you can't eat what's not there. After years of struggle, Joyce has lost 50 pounds and kept the weight off.

STEP 5. STRUCTURE AND ORGANIZE YOUR FOOD ENVIRONMENT

Structuring and organizing your food environment is vital for limiting the power of a bad boyfriend. Scheduling your meals and snacks and finding a regular time to exercise or even run errands can help structure your food environment. Also, plan your meals. It may seem boring, but know what you're having for breakfast, lunch, and dinner and for snacks. Don't go into food situations unprepared. You don't want to be scrambling when you're starving! Planning helps you resist temptation, especially the temptation of a bad boyfriend.

STEP 6. GUARD YOUR FOOD ENVIRONMENT

You know what they say: out of sight, out of mind! Do everything you can to keep your bad boyfriend out of your house, especially your kitchen. Unless it's for a special occasion and you feel confident that you can control your eating, avoid tempting food establishments such as ice cream stores or the corner bakery. Why set yourself up for failure?

In a groundbreaking study published in the *Journal of Neurosci-*

ence, researchers found a connection between brain responses to appetite-driven cues and future behavior. The first step toward controlling your cravings seems to be coming to an awareness of how much you're affected by specific triggers in the environment, such as the arrival of the dessert tray in a restaurant. Said the study's lead author, William Kelley, "You need to actively be thinking about the behavior you want to control in order to regulate it." In other words, use your head! You have to make a concerted effort to avoid the bad boyfriend drama.

Step 7. It Starts in the Cart

Want to know the number-one way to dump a bad boyfriend? Don't buy it in the first place. The first and most effective place to wash a bad boyfriend out of your hair is in the shopping cart. If you don't buy a bad boyfriend, you can't bring it into your house or office. Is there a better way to keep a bad boyfriend out of sight and out of mind? Remember that good fences make good neighbors. You can't have an illicit affair with someone who's not there.

My client Lori has been able to maintain her hard-earned weight loss by following the "smart cart" rule. "I shop very smart. If all that's in the fridge are apples and yogurt, then that's what I'll eat. But if I know there's a few boxes of Thin Mint Cookies in the house, I'll work on them until they're gone," she says. Lori controls her food environment with portion-controlled alternatives to her boyfriends, including 100-calorie bags of baked potato chips. Lori doesn't deprive herself, but she's always in control when it comes to her bad boyfriends.

Step 8. Learn from Your Past

All dieters must come to terms with their past attempts to control their weight, which probably included a fair share of disasters. You can look at your past efforts as failure, or you can learn from your mistakes. A child who's potty-training rarely succeeds on the first go-round. There are going to be a lot of misses and messes. Losing weight is no different. Expect setbacks, and anticipate failure. They're normal. But with each attempt, look at what works and what doesn't. The only way you ever really blow it is by not learning something from the experience. All mistakes are opportunities.

One way to make the transition from failure to success is to write down a list of your past attempts at losing weight. See what's worked for you and what's worked against you. This is critical. As we say in the world of dieting, "Those who fail to remember the past are condemned to wear it."

Here are some examples that a client shared with me:

What Works	What Doesn't
• Writing down what I eat	• Liquid meal replacements
• Carrying a piece of fruit in my bag every day	• Swearing off all starches
• Batch-cooking roasted vegetables	• Eating late at night
• Bringing lunch to work	• Skipping breakfast

Step 9. Plan, Prep, and Schlep

I have a favorite three-finger rule for breaking the boyfriend habit: *plan, prep, and schlep*. It may seem like a lot of work, but a little preparation can go a long way. To this day, I carry a food tote or refrigerated bag with me at all times. (And there are some cute ones out there!) Some clients keep a healthy food stash in their glove compartment or handbag. If you're planning on dining out, check the menu online beforehand and choose your meal before you're there and temptation sets in. Along those lines, you may want to eat something before heading out to a favorite restaurant. I can't tell you how many dieters deprive themselves of food all day and then go out to eat when they're starving. It's like Shark Week out there. It's a recipe for disaster! Eating when you're super-hungry all but guarantees that you'll overeat. The smartest girls I know have a light snack before heading out for a meal.

Step 10. Find a Nice Guy!

For every naughty boy who drives us to distraction, there's a great guy we'd be happy to take home to Mother. In the world of food, there are thousands of alternatives to the high-calorie, high-fat foods that keep doing us in. Consider a few nice guys that even your parents would approve of:

Bad Boys	Good Guys
• **Reduced-fat peanut butter**	• Better' n Peanut Butter • Justin's All Natural Peanut Butter (80-calorie individual packets) • Powdered peanut butter (such as PB2)
• **High-calorie, salty, crunchy snacks**	• 94% fat-free 100-calorie mini-bags of microwave popcorn • Individual portion-size bags of Popchips, Glenny's Soy Crisps, Glenny's Spud Delites, or Cape Cod 40% Reduced Fat Potato Chips • 100-calorie bag of pretzels, chips, or rice cakes • KA-ME rice crakers
• **Baked Goods**	• Individual packs of Skinny Cow, Weight Watchers, or Breyers frozen novelties (80-150 calories each) • Low-calorie double chocolate mousse! • Individually wrapped Fiber One brownies (100 calories each, with fiber) • Chocolite chocolate protein bars (60–120 calories each)

- Trader Joe's 100-calorie milk or dark chocolate bars
- NuGo Slim Brownie Crunch Bars (190 calories per bar)

- **Regular or whole-wheat pasta**
  - Nasoya Pasta Zero Plus (an entire 8-ounce bag has only 40 calories and looks just like pasta)
  - Fiber Gourmet Light Pasta (with the taste and texture of traditional pasta but 40 percent fewer calories—130 versus 210 per 2-ounce serving—this pasta's secret ingredient is a wheat-resistant starch)

- **Bagels**
  - Kim's Light Bagels or Western Bagel Alternative (many flavors, and only 110 calories per bagel)
  - Pepperidge Farm Bagel Flats (100 calories per flat)

- **Wraps/lavash (240 calories each)**
  - La Tortilla Factory Low Carb, High-Fiber Wraps (110 calories each)
  - Joseph's Flax, Oat Bran, and Whole Wheat Lavash Bread (100 calories per huge lavash)

- **Artisan breads**

- Flatout Foldit Flatbreads (60–120 calories each)

- **English muffins**

  "Lite" 100-calorie, high-fiber English muffins

The End of an Affair

WHY DO WE HANG IN WITH THESE BAD BOYFRIEND FOODS EVEN when every fiber of our being, not to mention our scales and waistlines, tells us they aren't the right fit?

Just like our real-life bad boyfriends, we enter into these relationships with heavy expectations. We spend countless hours and a lot of energy thinking about how we can work them into our lives. Like the handsome Lothario we make excuses for, or the multiple offender who showers us with blinding bling, certain foods make us do everything possible to make them a good match. How many times have you caught yourself saying, "It's okay. I'll have just a bite of cake or a handful of potato chips"?

In fact, this wouldn't be a problem at all if you could limit yourself to a single bite or handful. In the clear light of day, if you look at all of the time, energy, money, and aggravation your bad boyfriend food has cost you, then you'll soon come to the realization that this is a relationship that just won't work. It's a moment's pleasure for a lifetime of misery. Honestly, is there a food worth eating that constantly causes you to feel out of control, makes you do bad things, and damages your self-esteem?

It's time to grow up in the world of food. With the right strategies, nearly anyone can muster the strength and courage needed to say "good riddance" to a bad boyfriend food. Just like our romantic relationships, a healthy food relationship should be based on self-love and acceptance. It should fuel our self-esteem and allow us to thrive and feel happy.

Maya Angelou once said, "When you know better, you do better." The better you know the foods that work for you and the foods that work against you, the sooner you can stop obsessing and start living in the world of food. A healthy relationship with food doesn't have to involve sacrifice and denial. However, it does involve knowing the right tricks, tips, and alternatives so that food doesn't rule you. You are the queen of your castle, and you will rule the food.

CHAPTER 2

What Do the "It Girls" Know?

IF YOU'VE EVER HAD A BAD BOYFRIEND (AND IF YOU'RE READING this book, you've probably lost count), then you probably have a laundry list of guys you should have dumped and an even longer list of guys you wish you'd never even met. Some girls spend years in the "perfect" relationship only to find out that they should've been more on the ball from the beginning. It's amazing that millions of women settle for a guy even when their intuition tells them he's so wrong. Could you imagine walking into a store, seeing a beautiful couture gown with a huge stain on the sleeve, and thinking, *Well, aside from the stain, it's perfect. I'll just clean it at home.* Hello? Most of us wouldn't dare. But when it comes to men, we don't think twice about taking home a project—usually the one most desperately in need of fixing.

There are a select few women who manage to avoid all the nonsense. They can spot a bad boyfriend a mile away. At the first sign of trouble, they always cut and run. Their B.S. meter is forever on high alert, and they know all the red flags. No matter how great or tempting the package, they manage to steer clear of the bad boyfriends. It's "sayonara" to the dude who doesn't hold the door, bring flowers, or walk them to the front door. These gutsy girls don't measure guys by their looks, bank account, or charm. They don't do drama or get their hearts broken. They're never up late, staring into an empty carton of Häagen-Dazs mint chocolate chip and wondering if he'll call (or beating themselves up if he doesn't). To borrow a line from Rodgers and Hammerstein, they know how to wash that man right out of their hair.

Of course, these girls are definitely the exception, not the rule. They're the elite: a small group of take-no-crap It Girls who somehow manage to avoid the bad boyfriend trap. We admire these babes. We think, *How'd they pull that off, while we keep falling in the same hole, repeating the same behavior again and again? Are they blessed with magical powers? What's their secret?*

The Secret

WHEN IT COMES TO DIETING, THE IT GIRLS HAVE A CLEAR PLAN. IN a country where nearly 70 percent of dieters regain all the weight they lose within a year and 95 percent gain it all back within five years, these girls manage to lose weight and, more important, keep it off. Some never even struggle with their weight. They're slim and manage to stay that way.

In the world of dieting, these are the elite 5 percent. As in love, these girls never rely on willpower. An iron will never helped anyone stare down a box of Mallomars, say no to a plate of French fries, or fit into skinny jeans. The elite 5 percent go into every food situation with a powerful plan. They know what they want, and their expectations are high, but only because they know what to look out for. Every time they sit down to a meal or a snack, they have a list of bad boyfriends indelibly etched in their minds. They know the foods that do and don't work for their weight and their waistline. Foods that don't measure up aren't even given the time of day. For these girls, being thin and having a new pair of skinny jeans is a much better reward than the momentary pleasure of a cookie, candy bar, or glazed doughnut. They always keep their goals in sight, and they don't compromise.

Contrary to what you may think, these girls aren't smarter than you. But they know their own vulnerability, and they never lose sight of it. Never giving themselves the benefit of the doubt, they're very good at brutal self-assessment and truthful self-talk. They're not afraid to look in the mirror and say, *I can't even be around this food.*

I have one client for whom bread is a bad boyfriend. She can't even be near it. Just the sight and smell of a freshly baked baguette or roll triggers out-of-control cravings. As an executive headhunter, she regularly entertains clients at fancy restaurants. Instead of relying on a healthy dose of good fortune to avoid polishing off five rolls before the meal even arrives, she'll ask the waiter not to bring the bread basket. If her clients want bread, she'll request that the waiter take the bread away after they've made a selection. Bread is one of her bad boyfriends, and she knows it. On the other hand, this same client can take one or two bites of a French fry or a single spoonful of mashed potatoes and not even think twice about it. Unlike bread, potatoes aren't her bad boyfriends—they don't trigger her cravings and out-of-control eating. Some of us are attracted to the clean-shaven all-American guy; others go for the swarthy brunet with the slightly dimpled chin. What doesn't work for one may work for another. Whatever their preference, the elite 5 percent of girls know their bad boyfriends and realize that most of the time it's better not to get involved in the first place.

Now in my 16th year in the "it girl" ranks, I am proud to say that I live by the bad boyfriend rule. Recently, my son asked me to bake cupcakes for his eighth birthday. My little man must have come across one too many Betty Crocker wannabe moms while on playdates. My son is the love of my life, but I've never made cupcakes for this boy. The scent and sight of raw batter sends me into a tizzy. Batter is my Achilles' heel—a very, very bad boyfriend. If I tried to make cupcakes, half the batter would never make it into the muffin pan. I have a dysfunctional relationship with batter; it always gets the best of me. It lures me in, breaks my heart, and leaves me fat, guilty, and unhappy—every time!

Of course, I didn't want to disappoint my son or see him humiliated in front of his friends because of his mommy's issues with baked goods. How did I solve this bad boyfriend dilemma? I looked at my son's adorable face and told him that while Mommy doesn't make cupcakes, I can buy them from the store and bring them to his school. He could also have his personal favorite, Devil Dogs, which come individually wrapped and aren't even that tempting to me. For some reason, I can buy but I can't bake. Problem solved.

This is how the It Girls do it. They come into every food situation with a plan of attack. In my case, buying was the perfect alternative to baking. For years I was one of the millions of people in the country caught in the destructive cycle of losing and gaining back weight. I broke through—not by offering a sacrifice to the diet gods, but simply by developing strategies for avoiding the path that has always led me to gain weight. The good news is that you can join the ranks of the elite 5 percent. I'll show you how.

Keep Your Bad Boyfriends in Mind

IF YOU TRULY ASPIRE TO BE AN "IT GIRL," THE FIRST THING YOU'VE got to do is change your thinking. It can't be repeated often enough: being overweight isn't the problem. Being overweight is a symptom—a symptom of being out of control with food. Being overweight is a disease of thinking—"fat thinking" is what I like to call it. When it comes to dieting, our minds conspire against us. We think that going to the gym is a license to eat anything we want. We believe—and nearly every diet book and weight loss program I can think of counsels people—that it is possible to eat any food in moderation. Or that eating earlier in the day is better for our weight than eating at night. Few of us realize that food, our bad boyfriend food in particular, plays havoc with our sensitive neurochemistry.

In chapter 1, I mentioned the importance of knowing your bad boyfriend foods. Once you've committed your bad boyfriends to paper, things get a lot easier, since most of us have only a few foods that cause us to lose control. For the most part, it's better to keep these foods out of our homes, out of our environments, and out of our lives. If doughnuts are a bad boyfriend, then try to avoid situations that bring them into your food environment. That means taking a detour and going to the local coffeehouse for your coffee—not the convenient doughnut shop—or better still, having your coffee at home or bringing it with you if you have somewhere to go. It also means refraining from buying apple cider doughnuts—just for the car ride home—when you go apple-picking with the kids.

If things still aren't going well and you keep bumping into Mr. Wrong, think of the costs of this behavior.

- He's probably making your life miserable.
- He's probably robbing you of your dream of being skinny.
- He's disrupting your natural vibrancy and peace of mind.
- He's ruining your face and figure, as well as how you look and feel in your most gorgeous clothes.
- He's destroying your health or otherwise distracting you from the business of living.

It's worth *everything* to break the bad boyfriend habit! Life is short. Don't waste time with foods that prevent you from having the body and the life that you want.

It Girls Don't Do Moderation

Pick up any diet book and you'll see one universal piece of advice: "You can have anything in moderation." According to these books, no food is bad or off limits provided we don't eat too much of it. This is the one piece of "advice"—a term I use loosely—that has crushed the hopes and skinny dreams of more dieters than any other advice I can think of. I realize my comment stands in contrast to nearly everything you've ever heard about dieting. But people who can eat moderately or "sensibly," as one best-selling diet book author put it, don't need to diet. Let's get real, ladies. *If you could eat in moderation, you wouldn't have bought this book!*

In the philosophy of these wrongheaded diet plans, a dieting woman can eat a little of anything she wants. Hello? Can you imagine Carrie Bradshaw buying just one pair of heels at a Manolo Blahnik sample sale? Better yet, imagine having "moderate" sex on your honeymoon, or eating a "moderate" amount of cake on your birthday. If it feels good—and few things feel better than swan-diving into a bag of Hershey's Kisses or inhaling a box of Samoas—then we're going to do it to excess.

I have a client who's admitted to me on more than one occasion that she prefers the company of a bad boyfriend food to sex any day of the week. Putting aside the state of her personal life, my client was simply admitting to a reality of human behavior. Moderation seldom enters the equation when it comes to pleasurable activities like eating. How many "moderate" drug addicts do you know? I understand this is an extreme example, but there are similarities between drug and food addictions, as we'll learn in the next chapter. Simply stated, moderation doesn't work for a majority of dieters.

But that hasn't stopped experts from preaching moderation from the diet pulpit. Even the esteemed American Dietetic Association has gotten into the act. "All foods can fit into a healthful diet 'if' consumed in moderation with appropriate portion size and combined with regular physical activity." "*If* consumed in moderation"? Excuse me, but I think we need a reality check. Nearly 70 percent of adult Americans are overweight or medically obese. (If trends continue, that number is expected to hit 80 percent by 2030.) How many of these people pay attention to appropriate portion sizes? Or even exercise, for that matter?

In the last decade, portion sizes have expanded more than Victoria Beckham's wardrobe. In fact, serving sizes have grown over the past 20 years not only at fast-food places but also at other restaurants and even in our homes, according to a study in the prestigious *Journal of the American Medical Association*. It seems that the more we're given, the more we eat, a fact confirmed by Barbara Rolls, a leading researcher in the study of human eating behavior and the author of several best-selling diet books, including *The Ultimate Volumetrics Diet*. In a study published in the *American Journal of Clinical Nutrition,* Dr. Rolls and her colleagues gave volunteers varying amounts of macaroni and cheese each day for lunch. They wanted to see if larger portions led to greater consumption. The researchers found across the board that everyone responded to the increased portion size by eating more.

Not only are we not consuming foods in moderation, but a whopping 80 percent of adult Americans do not meet even the minimum daily recommendations for physical activity. And I would expect that number to be much higher among overweight adults. This is why concepts like "all foods fit" or "all foods in moderation" are a pipe dream for a majority of this country's 108 million active dieters.

Indeed, it's my view that words like "moderation" should be stricken from all discussions on weight control, despite our best efforts at rationalization (something most of us excel at, especially when it comes to bad boyfriends, not to mention bad boyfriend foods). If a food is a bad boyfriend, it's a safe bet that we'll never be able to enjoy it in moderation. Go back and look at your long-term relationship with food. How many times have you attempted to unsuccessfully control a certain food? How many times have these attempts led you right back to weight gain? How many times has overeating cookies, cake, or ice cream ruined your life and caused you to lose your mind? If cookies are your bad boyfriend, have you ever been able to eat them in moderation? The answer is almost certainly "no."

Counseling people to eat right or consume "healthier" foods isn't the answer either. Dieters aren't dummies. You'd be hard-pressed to find anyone in this country who still thinks Twinkies or French fries are even remotely healthy foods. Yet we consume these and thousands of other "unhealthy" foods at alarming rates while virtually ignoring healthy options such as fruits, vegetables, whole grains, and lean proteins. If we appeal exclusively to health, most people just continue to gain more and more weight. As Thomas Frieden, director of the U.S. Centers for Disease Control and Prevention, said recently, "Exhorting people to eat less and exercise more is totally ineffectual."

Again, it all goes back to our thinking. Here's an all too familiar scenario I encounter with my clients. After months of dieting, a client sees the scale drop to the number she's been targeting. Like clockwork, she cancels her next appointment and tells me she's feeling great and is "good to go." It can take a month, six months, or even a year, but nearly all clients who leave like this will regain every pound they lose. I can't tell you how many times I've been on the receiving end of an anguished phone call that starts something like this: "Lyssa, I gained back all of the weight you helped me lose. I feel awful. I was doing so well. How did this happen to me?"

How Did This Happen?

DO YOU REMEMBER TRAINING REALLY HARD AS A KID FOR A GYM-nastics meet or a ballet recital? You may have spent hundreds of hours on the beam or at the barre, perfecting your technique. This isn't unusual. Anything worthwhile takes time and dedication to master. The moment you stopped practicing, your skills probably went downhill.

Losing weight is no different. The It Girls put in a lot of time and effort building good habits. Losing weight and staying slim isn't just about eating the right foods in the right amounts. It's about building and continually practicing good habits, not just in the area of your weight but in all areas of your life. Those who manage their stress, get enough sleep, and enjoy healthy, loving relationships have an easier time losing weight and keeping it off. While this may seem like a lot to handle, especially when dealing with all of life's other headaches, it's nothing compared to the pain of being overweight, feeling unhappy, and forever careening out of control with food.

Joining the It Girl Ranks

NOW THAT YOU KNOW WHAT THE IT GIRLS DO (AND DON'T DO), how do you become one of them? Here's how you join the ranks.

1. **Be mature**. Act like the grown-up you are. It's time to abandon the childhood thinking that a chocolate chip cookie or bag of potato chips is a treat or reward. These foods may have been a reward when you were a little girl with a little girl's metabolism, but now you're a woman, with a woman's metabolism and a Louis Vuitton–size collection of emotional food baggage.

2. **Be selfish.** When it comes to losing weight, don't be afraid to speak up. I have a client who has an issue with pizza. She recently went to a friend's house for the weekend, and pizza was on the menu. She was too embarrassed to ask her host to serve something else, so she ate the pizza—and not just one slice, but half a pie. Pizza is her bad boyfriend, so this was entirely predictable. I told my client, as I tell everyone who comes to see me, that when it comes to your weight control efforts, you can't be afraid to speak up. My client should have said, "Thanks for the pizza, but this isn't good for me. Do you have anything else?"

   You need to work on yourself first and foremost. If

you're going out to dinner, don't be afraid to bring your own salad dressing, and don't spend time worrying what your dining companions will think if you instruct the waiter not to bring the bread basket to the table. Don't be too concerned with how any of this comes across to others. This is your weight and your life. No one else has to live it or fit into your pants but you.

3. **Know that time makes it easier.** Just because the weight is dropping off doesn't mean that the problem isn't there. I can get you to lose 10 pounds in 10 days. I really can. But changing your brain is going to take a little longer. The thinking that made you fat doesn't go away as the pounds drop off. But it will get easier with time.

4. **Expect some ups and downs**. Watching the numbers on the scale go down is a big turn-on. At those moments, you'll feel on top of the world. But sometimes the scale plateaus, your girlfriends stop gushing about how good you look, or you're faced with a few days of temptation that set you back. Stay focused, reignite your motivation, and don't let it stop you.

5. **Just let it go.** It's amazing how easily we forgive others but not ourselves. I have a friend who says that no one needs enemies because we're all our own worst enemies. When it comes to losing weight, don't expect perfection. Expect to fall off the wagon—expect to blow it. But forgive yourself, learn from your mistake, and move on. As I tell my clients,

"All-or-nothing thinking always leads to all-or-nothing eating."

6. **Understand that things change.** Did you know that palm trees bend but don't break? They can bend all the way to the ground during a hurricane, and when the storm is over they straighten up again and are actually stronger. In short, they're flexible. To succeed at losing weight and keeping it off, you have to be like a palm tree. What works at one point in time may not work at another.

   I have a client, Barbara, whose children were headed off to sleepaway camp. During the school year Barbara served dinner at 6:00 p.m. on the dot. With her kids away at camp for six weeks, things would be different. Her life was going to change, and so would her food life. What worked during the school year might not work during the summer. Barbara was going to have a lot of unstructured time, and unstructured time is the devil's harlot. She had to figure out a new way to structure her eating. With her kids away, Barbara knew she wouldn't be sitting down to dinner at night until around 8:00 p.m., when her husband got home from the office. She made sure to schedule a daily late afternoon snack that she had to have no later than 4:30 p.m. The lesson Barbara learned? Be flexible if a situation changes.

7. **Talk to yourself with respect and kindness.** We've all got one: an internal voice that offers opinions and then determines how we perceive every situation and

circumstance in our lives. When that voice is favorable, it lifts our self-esteem and self-image. When that voice is judgmental, it often engages in negative self-talk. Dieters are the worst offenders when it comes to negative self-talk. How often do you hear a girl at the next table lamenting, after polishing off the last piece of chocolate cake, that she "blew it"? This negative self-talk creates a self-fulfilling prophecy. Suddenly we stop looking for solutions and assume all is lost. "I've been fat my whole life. I might as well eat what I want." Instead of looking for solutions, we tell ourselves that we can't handle the challenges ahead.

This sort of self-sabotage is the Achilles' heel of most dieters. It Girls know how to do away with the internal negative dialogue. They know that a slipup doesn't have to be a life sentence. Learning to dispute negative self-talk takes time, but is worth the effort. In time, dieters are often surprised to discover that much of their negative thinking is inaccurate and exaggerated.

8. **Be authentic.** If you want to lose weight, personalize it to your own food life. As we learned in chapter 1, each of us has a long and sordid history with at least one bad boyfriend food that has constantly thwarted our efforts to fit into the latest fashions. Whatever diet you follow, it's got to be authentic to you and your unique relationship with food.

9. **Eat your water.** In an ideal world, (nonfried) vegetables should make up 50 to 60 percent of your daily calories.

In fact, they should take up the most real estate on your plate! Having said that, I also live in the real world. It's one thing to tell you to eat tons of vegetables, and it's another thing to get you to do it. I can lead you to a designer sample sale, but I can't force you to buy. If you're one of those girls who don't like vegetables, get creative. Try using pureed vegetables in sauces, sneaking them into burger patties, or finding some recipes that will work for you. I provide some great ones at the end of this book!

10. **If you bite it, write it**. I encourage all my clients to keep a detailed account of everything they put in their mouths, whether they scribble it on a pad or type it electronically. A food diary shows you exactly what you eat. You probably think that you know exactly what you eat every day. You probably even think you could guess the number of calories that you eat every day. But the truth is that most people eat more often and take in more calories than they think they do. Also, keeping track of your food over time will actually make you want to eat better. Every time you write down a food that has a lot of calories in it, you'll want to avoid it in the future. Your food diary can actually help you to look at food in a whole new way.

Beating the House

THERE'S A POPULAR SAYING IN GAMBLING CIRCLES, "THE HOUSE always wins." Yet millions of people willingly gamble away their hard-earned money, seduced by the delusion that if they keep at it long enough they'll win the "big one."

I always tell clients that in the world of food the house always wins. If you've spent your whole life duking it out with chocolate chip cookies, then you're unlikely to start winning that fight. Just as an emotional jolt compels a gambler to keep betting, millions of girls convince themselves that this go-round with a bad boyfriend food will be different. It's a lie, of course, but one impervious to any statistical argument against it.

It Girls have perspective. Memories of that one night of hot sex with a bad boyfriend fade fast. Just as they want and expect more from a romantic relationship, they want and expect more from a relationship with food. It Girls know that a moment's pleasure from a cookie, chocolate bar, or plate of fries can't compare to a lifetime of being in control of their eating, their weight, and their clothing size. As you read this book I think you'll discover that constantly betting on your weight and forever failing at dieting is much harder than resisting the temptation of a bad boyfriend food. Remember, food isn't a reward, treat, or trophy. There is no lotto jackpot in the world of food. The real prize is feeling happy because food is no longer the overlord of your life.

CHAPTER 3

Love at First Bite: Food and Your Brain

A S A TOP CORPORATE ATTORNEY AND MOTHER OF TWO RAM-bunctious boys, Rachel has always thought of herself as one tough cookie. Willpower and perseverance are her constant companions. She worked her way through law school, graduating near the top of her class. She was the youngest person in her firm to make partner. At age 35, she completed her first triathlon after the birth of her second son. "No obstacle is too great," she's fond of telling her boys.

So you can imagine how disheartening it was for Rachel to struggle to control her appetite for creamy, sweet frozen treats. Rachel's ice cream habit had started innocently enough. "It was a nice way to end my day," she explained to me during our first consultation. Before too long, the half-cup-serving-size bowl she purchased just to limit her overconsumption of ice cream was being filled five times a night. Eventually, Rachel just did away with the serving bowl and started eating right out of the carton. Rachel may have been a tough cookie, but when it came to ice cream, she was strictly Mrs. Softy.

Rachel's story isn't uncommon. Like many dieters, she had the best intentions and was determined to take her place among the ranks of the It Girls. How was it possible that "a nice way to end the day" ended up as 15 extra pounds? Sitting in my office, Rachel called herself "weak" and "stupid." In every area of her life, Rachel had used an iron will to succeed, even against seemingly insurmountable odds. Now, here she was: partner in a blue-chip law firm, wife, mother of two, and accomplished amateur triathlete knocked senseless by a carton of mint chocolate chip ice cream.

If you find yourself, like Rachel, getting weak in the knees around ice cream or any number of sinfully rich, creamy desserts on a regular basis, the good news is that you're not entirely to blame. In recent years, a whole new field of scientific research has emerged to explain why for most of us it's hard, if not impossible, to just say no to food. Cravings for sweet, salty, and crunchy foods—almost invariably our bad boyfriends—are similar to substance abuse and other more commonly recognized addictions in their course and action.

The very thought that a doughnut, cookie, or potato chip could be as addictive as drugs would have seemed laughable to scientists just a few years ago. We now know different. Since the mid-1990s, there's been a steady rise in research on food addiction and the chemistry of weight gain. It's now well established that many of our favorite bad boyfriend foods, such as cookies, chips, and French fries, hijack the brain's reward center in much the same way that cocaine, alcohol, nicotine, and other highly addictive substances do. Brain scans of obese people and compulsive eaters reveal major league disturbances in the brain's reward circuits that are strikingly similar to those experienced by drug addicts. This is just the tip of the iceberg.

Marcel Proust, Food Scientist

AUTHOR MARCEL PROUST MEMORABLY TAPPED INTO THE FACT
that food has the ability to wreak havoc with our sensitive neurochemistry. In 1913, Proust's favorite cookie, the madeleine, now available
at every Starbucks counter, inspired a seven-volume literary masterpiece, *Remembrance of Things Past*. As Proust recalls:

> No sooner had the warm liquid mixed with the crumbs touched
> my palate than a shudder ran through me and I stopped, intent
> upon the extraordinary thing that was happening to me. An ex-
> quisite pleasure had invaded my senses, something isolated, de-
> tached, with no suggestion of its origin. . . . The taste was that of
> the little piece of madeleine which on Sunday mornings at Com-
> bray (because on those mornings I did not go out before mass),
> when I went to say good morning to her in her bedroom, my aunt
> Léonie used to give me, dipping it first in her own cup of tea or
> tisane. The sight of the little madeleine had recalled nothing to
> my mind before I tasted it. And all from my cup of tea.

Notice that Proust says that just a taste of a favorite childhood treat
gave rise to a surge of craving memories. One hundred and fifty years
before there was even remote scientific knowledge of the effect of food
on our bodies and minds, Proust described the power and truth of in-
voluntary memory.

Proust's favorite childhood treat revealed a past lying dormant
within him, ready to be called back to consciousness. This recollection
was triggered by the physical sensation of biting into a cookie. "It is a
complete fragment of the past, with its original 'perfume,' that is for a
moment given back to us," he said.

The physiology of Proust's *petite madeleine* experience is well understood by science. The olfactory (smell) system, for instance, has a direct, primitive connection to a region of the brain known as the hypothalamus. This connection gives certain odors a special power to trigger memories in some detail. I have a client who tells me that she can't walk by a pizza parlor without recalling Sunday dinners at her grandmother's house.

Food Stimuli: Why "Feasting with Your Eyes" Isn't Just a Saying

OUR BODIES ARE SMART, BUT THEY GET CONFUSED FROM TIME TO time. I counsel clients to keep their bad boyfriend foods out of sight. This is because the cravings don't start in your stomach. Often a craving begins with a longing glance—like the steamy gaze the spoiled daughters in those Spanish-language telenovelas are always throwing at the shirtless gardeners.

It's true: eating starts with your eyes. Just looking at appetizing food can make you hungry! An important study by leading researchers at the prestigious Max Planck Institute of Psychiatry found that the production of a primary hunger hormone, ghrelin, increases after simply looking at pictures of food. These same studies show that in addition to the physiological factors that get your body the calories it needs, environmental factors also have a very real influence on which foods you eat and how much. So when savvy advertisers show tempting, mouthwatering treats on TV, when your coworker keeps a sugary candy jar on her desk, or when you leave food out on your kitchen counter, you'll eat with your eyes and then see the damage on your thighs.

Smelling foods we crave works the same way. Ever walk by a bakery and suddenly feel hungry? Even if you just had a big meal, you may find yourself stopping for a favorite treat. My client Susan learned this lesson the hard way. She left her five-year-old son's birthday cake out on the counter after his party. Of course, she had ordered her favorite from the most popular bakery in town: vanilla cake with chocolate frosting. The party was over, and half the cake stood uneaten. She decided to save it, reasoning that her son and husband would polish it off.

As she prepped dinner the next day Susan started slowly cutting off slivers of slices to make the lines on the cake straight. *Stop it,* she told herself. But whenever she glanced at the cake she would cut away another slice. In no time the cake was gone and Susan was left with self-loathing, shame, and a slightly distended belly. When her son asked for a slice of his birthday cake after he finished his dinner, Susan burst into tears.

Susan's story is a familiar one. Every day thousands of dieters fall prey to the power of seductive visuals. In another study, researchers at the Max Planck Institute showed test subjects images of either delicious food or non-edible objects. Then they measured levels of different hunger hormones in their blood, such as ghrelin, an appetite stimulator, and insulin and leptin, which are appetite suppressors. The researchers observed that the amount of ghrelin in the blood actually increased specifically in response to the enticing food images. Simply seeing food involuntarily triggers our appetite, which explains why Susan sliced and diced her way through her son's birthday cake.

The Demon Binger

PICTURE THIS SCENARIO: IT'S THREE O'CLOCK IN THE AFTERNOON, and you're home alone staring blankly into the vast space that is your refrigerator. You may start off easy. Perhaps you grab a few carrots, followed by a piece of leftover chicken and a bowl of cold pasta. Like a shark that smells blood in the water, your feeding frenzy accelerates. In no time flat you plow through crackers, peanut butter, and a granola bar. Then you move on to the pantry. Chips, cookies, frosting, stale Halloween candy—nothing is off limits. You feel possessed, like Linda Blair herself has taken over your body and mind. However, it's not a demon. It's the appetite-stimulating hormone neuropeptide Y, which was already hard at work when you started snacking and you unwittingly sent it into hyperdrive.

Why should you care about a hormone? High-fat and high-sugar foods stimulate the release of neuropeptide Y, which ignites appetite and causes us to gorge on whatever is within arm's reach. Since neuropeptide Y responds to fat and sugar, the more simple carbs you devour the more your brain tells you to keep chowing down.

Not eating for long periods of time (the body considers that anything more than four daytime hours) also increases neuropeptide Y production. When you finally do eat, you may stuff your face to compensate for earlier missed calories. If you're bingeing at the same time of the day, every day, you may be eating too few calories, which is why I tell clients that the best way to beat back cravings is to never to skip meals.

HOW TO BEAT OVEREATING

Do you find yourself rummaging through the pantry or caught in a face-off with the fridge? If this is your pattern, then you're setting yourself up for cravings. My client Wendy explains: "Since I work full-time, I scheduled my son's teacher conference during my lunch hour. I didn't have time to stop for lunch before going back to the office, so I grabbed a protein bar and coffee from the newsstand, hoping it would hold me over. The minute I walked in the door after work I made a beeline for the fridge without even bothering to take off my coat. In a flash, I was scooping peanut butter out of the jar. And that was just the beginning. By the time my husband came home and we sat down for dinner, I had plowed through half a box of cookies, two slices of pie, and two bowls of cereal. To top it all off, I still ate my dinner!"

Wendy had good intentions but was no match for neuropeptide Y. As your blood sugar dips and neuropeptide Y rises, it's critical to have a snack, especially one high in protein, in the midafternoon to help you get through the witching hour.

THE CRAZY THING ABOUT ANOREXIA

As an intern in graduate school, I frequently worked with people who were anorexic. One of the first things I learned about them blew me away: many are clinically obese. They often have higher body fat ratios than normal-range people of the same age. Looking at their stick-thin physiques, I wondered how this could be.

If you're starving or drastically cutting back on calories for long periods of time, your metabolism slows to a crawl and your body begins storing fat. A body in starvation or calorie-restriction mode runs through its carbohydrate calories first, then turns to its protein stores; lastly, it dips into its fat reserves.

The anorectic body allocates its precious carbohydrate and protein resources toward much-needed fuel, leaving nothing but fat behind. When we don't eat the right combinations of foods on a regular schedule, our hormonal reactions are beyond our control.

Feel Good Hormones: Friend or Foe?

You may have heard of dopamine. It's an amazing little neurotransmitter (a chemical responsible for ensuring proper communication between the brain's nerve cells) that's been studied for more than 60 years and is the subject of more than 100,000 scientific research papers. In the brain, dopamine neurons wear multiple hats (and some very fashionable ones at that). One of the best-described roles for dopamine neurons is in learning about rewards. In particular, dopamine neurons in an area of the brain called the ventral tegmental area (VTA) get aroused when something good happens unexpectedly, such as the sudden availability or expectation of sex or drugs. Many foods also trigger the release of VTA dopamine. Some of these are perfectly healthy choices, such as strawberries, blueberries, bananas, fish, or eggs. However, dopamine is also released in the presence of many unhealthy, high-calorie foods, thus contributing, some researchers believe, to their seemingly addictive properties.

Take sugar as an example. Our ability to sniff out calories in the form of cake, cookies, and candy depends on sugar's intoxicating effect on our brain's dopamine-rich reward center, an area known as the nucleus accumbens. Not coincidentally, the NA is the hub of reward activity for all addictive drugs.

In a breakthrough study, researchers at Duke University and the Universidade do Porto in Portugal demonstrated that genetically altered mice with an inability to taste sweet foods consistently chose sugar water, even though they couldn't sense the sugar. These findings, according to the researchers, suggest that calorie-rich nutrients "can directly influence brain reward circuits that control food intake independently of palatability or functional taste transduction." In other words, even if cake and cookies don't arouse your loins, and they're not in the bad boyfriend category, you could end up craving them anyway.

What's interesting about this study is that the sugar-blind mice didn't opt for the low-calorie sugar alternative, a mixture of water and sucralose otherwise known as Splenda. It seems that the artificial sweeteners don't provide the same dopamine boost along the brain's reward pathways as the real thing.

These finding shouldn't come as such a shock. Let's be honest, ladies: how many of you opt for a diet version of your favorite food when the higher-calorie bad boy is staring you in the face? If you're like me and you've plowed through a tub of Ben & Jerry's or a bowl of chocolate chip cookie dough in a single sitting, you know that the taste of these foods overrides your stomach's plea, "I'm so full I could hurl at any moment." That little reward signal in the brain supersedes everything else.

The freaky thing about eating high-calorie, bad boyfriend food is that not only does this food change our dress size and waistlines, but it also alters our brains. In another experiment, rats fed a steady diet of bad boyfriend foods got fat but had lower levels of dopamine in their brains than rats that dined on normal fare. How is this possible, you might ask, given that foods such as chocolate, processed cheese, and potato chips trigger the release of dopamine? According to researchers, yummy bad boyfriend foods change our brains by adding fuel to the fire. Being fat actually weakens the dopamine system, reducing the number of dopamine receptors in the brain and making it less sensitive to the satiety message. This is why people who are overweight don't get much reward from food and they just keep eating. It's a horrible cycle that has led to the new food nymphomaniacs.

Is Stress Making You Fat?

IT'S NOT YOUR IMAGINATION—STRESS REALLY CAN PACK ON THE pounds. How many times have you put your foot in your mouth? Well, in this case, it's food in your mouth. Do you spoon peanut butter out of the jar after you get your Visa bill? Do you fantasize about a Snickers bar after a dress-down by your boss? It's not that you're a lost cause. Stressful situations can create cravings for carbohydrate-rich snack foods, not simply because they taste good, but because they also calm the stress hormones adrenaline and CRH (corticotrophin-releasing hormone) cortisol. Eating makes us feel good, and certain foods, that are nutritionally barren and made up of mostly sugar, like desserts and simple carbohydrates, affect brain chemicals to improve mood. It's not usually a particular food you want, but rather the feeling of comfort and pleasure that food provides.

A common scenario is that a stressor (your mother-in-law, for instance) has upset the chemical balance in your brain (she's coming and there's nothing you can do about it), and your body wants you to do something about it to restore balance. This can make you very susceptible to emotional eating and trigger a desire for "comfort foods" (pass the pretzels, please). These foods aren't necessarily addictive, but they're just a quick and effective way to bring your stress hormones back down.

In the days of the caveman, stress gave us the extra energy (calories) to mobilize a response to life-or-death danger. Today we take our stress to the local pizzeria and eat it at the counter. These extra calories aren't used in battle, but rather, go straight to our hips. What to do? We need to find ways other than eating to stay calm, cool, and collected. We need tips and tricks that soothe us under stress and release feel-good chemicals in your brain.

NINE ANTI-STRESS STRATEGIES

1. **Choose a soothing alternative to eating.** Activities such as massage, music, talking to a friend, relaxation techniques, exercise, reading a good book, knitting, and yoga are great for reducing stress.

2. **Write it down.** Get stress off your mind and onto the page. The very act of doing this can be cathartic and give you a fresh perspective.

3. **Meditate.** It's known as a great way to relax, but meditation also is helpful for gaining the self-awareness and self-regulation needed to change your relationship with food and even control overeating.

4. **Go online.** Read blogs and join message boards or support groups. These things lend support and community, which can help you feel less alone and isolated. You'll understand that you're not the only one going through this experience, and you'll connect with others who are similarly struggling with their weight. It has a normalizing effect. That's why I often share my own weight loss journey with my clients—because I want them to know that I'm the same as they are.

5. **Breathe deeply.** Inhale through your nose, exhale through your mouth, and hold the breath for five seconds.

6. **Take inventory.** Look around and name the things near you. Taking notice of yourself in your physical space can center you immediately.

7. **Give yourself a reality check.** Ask yourself: Will this really matter one week, one month, or one year from now? Is there anything I can do right now to improve the way I'm feeling?

8. **Banish all-or-nothing negative thinking.** It's not too late to get back on the bandwagon with your food plan. If you mitigate damages, the less you have to lose later.

9. **Take small steps.** Write out a few ways in which you can break down this problem into manageable pieces. Action always feels better than inaction.

The Dieter's Dream: Sleep

LOSING WEIGHT WHILE YOU SLEEP SOUNDS LIKE A DIETER'S DREAM, but it's not! Getting the recommended eight hours of sleep each night actually curbs your appetite.

A team of researchers from the University of Chicago found that sleep deprivation upsets our hormonal balance, decreasing production of the appetite-suppressing hormone leptin, while increasing the production of the hunger hormone ghrelin. Ever have a sleepless night followed by a day of nonstop nibbling? Sleep deprivation tricks us into believing we're hungry even though we're not, so we eat. Retiring early can save you calories by keeping these hormones in check and keeping your appetite from getting stimulated. I advise clients to start unwinding at least an hour before lights out, which means no TV, radio, computer, phone, or i-anything!

Is Your Schedule Making You Fat?

DO YOU REMEMBER THE LAST TIME YOU SAT DOWN AND HAD A healthy meal with all the food groups represented? I didn't think so. These days, we're busier than ever. In fact, we're so busy that we're not eating right. Here are some of popular excuses I hear.

- "I'm too busy to stop and eat a 'real' lunch."
- "I'm too busy to pack a snack to bring with me."
- "I'm too busy to make dinner, so I'll just order takeout."
- "I'm too busy to go to the supermarket, so I'll just eat whatever is around the house."
- "I'm too busy to schlep, plan, and prep for tomorrow, so I'll just see where the day takes me."
- "I'm too busy to think about me."

Things have gotten so bad that we are no longer getting a majority of our calories from meals. As Michael Pollan observed in his best-selling book *Cooked: A Natural History of Transformation,* we now spend 78 minutes a day on secondary eating and drinking, more time than we give to meals, or primary eating, which is 67 minutes a day. Astoundingly, 20 percent of our food intake occurs in our cars. Secondary eating is now the new primary eating. And even when we do take time to sit down to meals, we gobble the wrong things, at the wrong times, upsetting our brains' delicate neurochemistry.

At one point or another, we've all fallen into the hectic schedule trap. No matter how busy you are, you always have to find time to eat. If you don't, even the skinniest skinny jeans won't fit you. Luckily, bad diet habits are meant to be broken. Here are 12 bad diet habits and the strategies needed to correct them.

Born to Be Broken: Top Bad Food Habits

Bad Habit #1: Eating Only When You're Hungry. If you've waited until you are physically hungry to eat, you've waited too long. That means your blood sugar has dropped and your neuropeptide Y is elevated. You're drastically increasing the chances of overeating because your body wants you to take in excess insulin in case you should decide to starve it again.

Correction: *Never eat when you're hungry.* Always eat before you get to the point of true hunger. Not sure what real hunger feels like? It feels awful—the shakes, irritability, tiredness, even some nausea.

Bad Habit #2: Cleaning Your Plate. The "clean your plate club" is one you *don't* want to be a member of. Some people have trouble leaving food behind when eating out. *We want our money's worth!* Better to throw some food out, however, than throw away your self-esteem, self-confidence, and lost pounds!

Correction: In a restaurant, when your food arrives, mark the amount you plan to eat by physically moving it over on your plate and ask to have the other half wrapped to go. That way you avoid the guilt of wasted food and stay true to your skinny jeans dream.

Bad Habit #3: Skipping Breakfast. Some of us are breakfast haters. We may think eating in the morning will make us hungrier. Or we reason that we don't have the time. Problem is that you've been fasting for eight to twelve hours, and if you don't eat anything in the morning, you literally have no fuel in the tank. Eventually your body stalls, and when it does, you'll reach for whatever is around.

Correction: Getting consensus among nutritionists is like getting consensus on the best way to achieve peace in the Middle East. But one thing the majority seems to agree on is the importance of breakfast. Diet champs eat breakfast, even if it's just a piece of whole wheat toast with jam or a glass of vegetable juice. Remember that breakfast is your first meal after several hours without eating. You don't have to force-feed yourself by a certain time in the morning, but I recommend that you eat before noon.

EASY BREAKFAST IDEAS

Not only do non-breakfast-eaters tend to eat more food at lunch and dinner and more snacks in between than their breakfast-eating girlfriends, but many studies indicate that eating fewer, larger meals each day causes body fat to increase more readily than consuming the same number of total calories over a series of smaller, more frequent meals. You don't have to eat a four-course meal in the morning; a little something will work here. Breakfast can be quick and portable (even made the night before) on the Skinny Jeans Diet—a peanut-butter-and-jelly sandwich or low-fat grilled cheese, a high-fiber, low-calorie muffin, or some fruit and yogurt. How about making a meal the whole family can enjoy, like high-protein eggs, whole-grain waffles, or high-fiber cereal?

You need fuel so that you can run around all morning doing whatever it is you do and so you don't eat more later. Eating breakfast is a secret of the elite 3 percent who lose weight and keep it off. It's easier and a lot more fun than starving until lunch.

Bad Habit #4: Eating on Cruise Control. Much of our daily eating happens on cruise control. Do you find your hand in the cereal box? Do you always grab a doughnut with your morning cup of coffee? Do you lick the last speck of batter from the bottom of the mixing bowl? These small habits can cause diet disaster. Picture all those bites, licks, and tastes going into a Ziploc bag. Now think about adding up those calories at the end of the day.

Correction: *Pay attention!* Pull yourself into the present, and be aware of how you feel, what you're putting into your body, and *why*. Make sure you know what you're doing—and remembering the consequences.

Bad Habit #5: Eating While Distracted. Eating in the car or while reading or watching television may cause you to lose track, leading to mindless grazing. Studies have found that people who are distracted while having a meal consume far more unhealthy snack food afterward than those who are paying close attention to what they eat. Even reading a book or having an animated discussion over a meal can have the same distracting effect.

Correction: Do you like to talk on the phone in the kitchen but end up with your hand in the cookie jar? Say hello, living room! Step into your living room—or whatever room you rarely go into, let alone eat in—for your phone conversations.

Bad Habit #6: Weekend Weight Gain. Did you ever have a great week of healthy eating followed by a calorie-laden weekend of barbecues, cocktail parties, and family dinners that put you firmly back at square one come Monday morning? We become altogether different people on weekends, consuming more booze and more calorie-dense foods than we do during the week. For most people, weekends are a recipe for diet disaster. One of the biggest dieting mistakes is going hungry all day to save your appetite for a fancy dinner, a party, or a big night on the town.

Correction: I always tell clients to eat something before a big event, such as a 100- to 150-calorie snack. A small snack ahead of time will limit overeating at the big event. Not only will eating before you go out lessen the likelihood of overeating, but it may also help slow you down when you finally do sit down to that celebratory meal. Studies have found that eating slowly helps your brain tell your stomach that it's had enough.

Bad Habit #7: Drinking Your Calories. Sugar-laden soda, alcohol, and fancy coffee drink calories add up.

Correction: Alcohol has a disinhibiting effect, which can cause you to overeat. The more you overeat, the less you pay attention to your diet, and you become less concerned about what you put in your mouth. Remember that liquid calories count just as much as solid calories, so everything you put in your mouth counts. I don't like to spend my calorie budget on liquids, but if this is your preference, consider any number of great-tasting, low-calorie alternatives such as a Skinny Chai Latte, fruit-flavored herb tea, or diet hot chocolate, such as Swiss Miss.

Bad Habit #8: Winging It. Planning can make or break a diet, but sometimes even the best of plans can go astray.

Correction: *Pack up for backup!* Carry a food bag with you. Bring a turkey sandwich just in case they don't serve lunch at the teacher meet-and-greet. Always keep some snacks on hand, just in case.

Bad Habit #9: Eating While Leaning . . . over the counter, kitchen sink, or open fridge.

Correction: Standing and eating doesn't register psychologically the way sitting and eating does. This results in nonstop noshing instead of a scheduled meal or snack. When it comes to eating habits, your fourth-grade teacher had it right: "Sit down and pay attention!"

Bad Habit #10: Failing to Plan Ahead. It's cliché but true. If you fail to plan, plan to fail.

Correction: One of my favorite tips: keep a bedside food journal to write down each night what you plan to eat the next day. By then, you pretty much know what the next day's schedule looks like, where you're having lunch, and what you plan to bring as snacks or assemble for dinner. Structuring tomorrow's eating instantly gives you a feeling of control over your food selections and eating schedule.

WHY MOST BOXED-MEAL DIETS ARE LIKELY TO FAIL

Did you know that boxed-meal diets have the highest weight rebound rate of any diet plans out there? That's because once you stop eating their food in a box, you gain the weight back, often with interest. You learn no strategies for your personal relationships with food when the food comes in a box. All you learn to do is open your wallet and spend a lot of money, then learn how long to microwave it. Instead of relying on boxed diets, do the work yourself and you'll get to your goal. It's amazing how a little planning goes such a long way. You'll be fitting into your clothes, feeling great, and looking hot. You worked it, so you earned it. All of it!

Bad Habit #11: Bargain Basement Shopping. Those wholesale clubs are no bargain for your waistline. When we buy huge amounts of food for our families, we then feel anxious about having all that food in the house. We can't throw it out, because that would be wasting money. So we eat it . . . which is the very thing we don't want to do! The big (no pun intended) problem now is a three-month supply of pretzels.

Correction: You're better off sticking to books and supplies at those wholesale clubs. Food bargains get calorically expensive very quickly.

Bad Habit #12: Keeping Meals Exciting. It may seem like a contradiction, but if you really want to lose that muffin top, don't keep your kitchen filled with four different kinds of cookies, chips, flavored rice cakes, ice cream, or other simple carbs—even if they are low-calorie. Think buffets and new restaurants—don't they cause you to fall apart? If you're like most of us, you do. *We eat more when there's variety.* As Tara Parker Pope stated in the *Wall Street Journal,* "Variety stimulates consumption." In a one-day study, people who were offered pasta in three different shapes ate 600 calories, but people who were offered pasta in one shape ate only 500.

    Correction: Embrace monotony. All successful diets, and all successful dieters, have a degree of monotony. It gives the dieter structure and routine and makes losing weight easier. Boring is the new best.

Why a Cookie Isn't Your Destiny

As a dietician, I've been privileged to help hundreds of people lose weight and forever change their thoughts and feelings about food. Perhaps the greatest of all rewards is seeing people rid themselves of shame and guilt and finally do away with the idea that they're weak or have some sort of disease just because they go weak in the knees around French fries, cookies, or dinner rolls. Many clients find it empowering to learn about how food affects their behavior.

    The new science of food and behavior points out why we need more than determination and the well-intentioned advice of our friends to overcome the seductive powers of our bad boyfriends. I'm confident that tips, tricks, and the strategies offered in this book can help you beat back the powerful influence of your bad boyfriend foods and finally take control of your life and dress size. Discovering the secrets to the seductive power of your bad boyfriends can help you make the big girl decision to either keep these foods in your life or let them go forever.

We may not be able to alter our biology. If you've always overeaten cookies, then this is probably something that will always be your issue. However, you can change the effect that cookies have on your life and waistline.

CHAPTER 4

Emotional Eating: The Food and Mood Connection

J ANE WASN'T WORRIED. AFTER ALL, SHE'D BEEN THROUGH this ritual three times before. The sadness, grief, and depression that overcome many parents after the kids leave home wasn't going to get the best of her. So when Jane's youngest daughter, Melissa, finally headed off to college, she told friends that having spent the better part of three decades focused on raising her children and caring for her home and family, she looked forward to a quiet house and some "me" time. It wasn't until a week later, while Jane was straightening up Melissa's room, that the reality of her newly empty nest hit her full force. Jane's husband, Peter, found her hours later sitting on the edge of Melissa's bed, sobbing uncontrollably.

In truth, Jane dreaded seeing her youngest child leave home. Peter tried to reassure her that Melissa's leaving was hardly the end—of being a parent or of her relationship with her daughters. These facts didn't matter to Jane. To soothe her distress and cope with the sadness and overwhelming anxiety she experienced over her family's changing dynamic, Jane turned to comfort food—and lots of it. Jane felt powerless over the circumstances of her life. She confided to Peter that she felt "useless" now that she no longer had children to care for.

Jane's feelings of powerlessness manifested themselves in food. Just a month after Melissa left home, Jane confessed that she couldn't stop eating. "Every day I try, and every day I give in to my urges to eat and eat. I'm hiding candy bars and bags of potato chips all over the house," she told me. At lunch with friends, Jane started indulging in the bread basket, something she'd studiously avoided for years. At night she'd often walk by Melissa's empty room and then make a beeline for the fridge, where she'd devour just about anything she could get her hands on. While grocery shopping, she found herself still buying food for a 17-year-old, three-varsity-sport daughter.

Jane's watershed moment came after Melissa returned from college for Thanksgiving break. Most students gain weight when they go off to college, but in this instance it wasn't Melissa who packed on the proverbial freshman 15. It was Jane.

Jane finally recognized that things had slipped beyond her control when the little black dress she bought for a charity event didn't make it past her thighs. I tell clients that tight clothing is the alarm bell for their weight, which is why buying only one size of clothing is a great strategy for helping keep weight off.

By the time Jane came to see me, it was clear that her eating was out of control. "How did this happen to me?" she asked. Deep down, Jane knew that she was eating to feed the loneliness and grief that she, like many parents, was experiencing because her daughter had left home. As I questioned Jane about her eating behavior, it became clear that unlike many "mood" eaters, she wasn't that discriminating with her food choices. Any small food that could be quickly popped into her mouth—cookies, mini-muffins, potato chips, pretzels, M&Ms—would suffice. It became clear that the bite-size snacks Jane was abusing were the same foods she used to buy for Melissa and her friends. After noting that Melissa had left for college in August and now it was November, I felt compelled to ask Jane: "Why are you still buying her snack foods and bringing them into the house?"

Jane knew she couldn't fill the void with food. She freely admitted that she'd fallen victim to emotional eating. Still, I reassured her that she didn't need a therapist. Jane's mood eating was more situational than psychological. It was triggered by empty nest syndrome. After reassuring Jane that her feelings were completely normal for someone who'd devoted the better part of her life to raising children, we came up with a plan for ending her mood eating as quickly as it began. We started with a simple trick I've used with hundreds of clients: a revised grocery list.

This new list had none of the snack foods that Jane used to buy for her children, including her personal bad boyfriend—ice cream. Once her bad boyfriend food and other snack foods were crossed off her shopping list, a funny thing happened: her mood eating disappeared and she lost weight. One of the most interesting things about emotional eating is that when the food isn't immediately available, even the most hardened eaters find a different outlet. Mood eaters are looking for immediate relief from their emotional condition, so they'll busy themselves with any convenient activity—even a non-eating one—

that distracts their attention. Scratching certain foods off Jane's shopping list and getting them out of the house did wonders for her life. I reassured her that no matter how terrible she might be feeling or how overwhelming her sadness might seem, she couldn't eat what wasn't within reach. When it comes to emotional eating, out of sight really is out of mind.

TO LIST OR NOT TO LIST

An interesting question was brought up to me recently in a session: What do you do if you don't like making or following a shopping list? My answer was simple. What do you do if you don't floss your teeth? Just as you'll get tooth decay and gum disease, if you don't follow a list, your diet will fall apart. A diet is a structured way of eating. Once you lift that structure, you're venturing out into the world of food much like a kid let loose in a candy store. If you're the typical American dieter who's making five weight-loss attempts a year, stuck on the diet merry-go-round, and you tell me you don't make a shopping list, I'm going to tell you to make a list. You need structure. Remember, skinny starts in the cart.

Just four months after our meeting, Jane had officially joined the ranks of the It Girls. She was 20 pounds lighter, and the little black dress was moving past her thighs with ease. Jane went beyond losing the freshman 15 by committing to a daily three-mile walk with her husband, which she confided was even better than ice cream.

What exercise did for Jane is the same thing a shopping list did for her: it gave her structure. As we'll see later on, exercise has limited value in helping people lose weight. But it's helpful for helping people keep weight off. Why? Exercise helped structure Jane's day. In time it became part of her routine, like brushing her teeth. Exercise gave Jane focus—a focus away from food and the emotional pain that had led her to gain weight. And by walking with her husband, exercise also made her accountable. She had to show up.

What Is Emotional Eating?

EMOTIONAL OR "MOOD" EATING IS THE BIG WHITE ELEPHANT IN the room. It afflicts millions of people and is the most common issue I see with clients. It's right there staring us in the face, causing havoc, and disrupting our lives. Rather than talking about our uncomfortable feelings or emotions, most of us would rather hide in a dish of ice cream, a bag of popcorn, or a slice of pizza.

Mood eating seldom has anything to do with food. Whether we're bored, worried, or lonely, food is an immediate, convenient way to divert attention from our emotional distress. At one time or another, we've all eaten in response to our feelings. Anxiety over an upcoming job interview may send you searching for the nearest bag of potato chips. A fight with your spouse may prompt an all-out ice cream binge.

A $2,000 fender-bender may send you fleeing to the nearest Dunkin Donuts. A bag of cookies might be the best way to ease your boredom. For many of us, our strongest food cravings seem to hit when we're at our weakest point emotionally. Bottom line: we seek comfort in food when emotional "hunger" strikes.

Strong emotions and feelings drive impulsive eating. Mood eaters want something that tastes good and can be quickly and easily popped into their mouths, such as a piece of candy or bite-sized cookie. These foods are often sweet or salty, crunchy or creamy. Though these bad boys are short in stature, they pack a powerful one-two punch. Studies show that the textures and tastes of our favorite bad boy foods provide immediate gratification. Food manufacturers know this. The packaging and advertising for sweet, salty, and crunchy snack foods are carefully designed to get you to buy and overconsume. Snack foods are an immediate, impersonal outlet that lets you spill your emotions without fear of reprisal or judgment.

My client Pam, a small-business owner and mother of two young girls, loves to cook for her family. But when she's flipping out, she doesn't prepare a three-course turkey dinner; she reaches for a bag of potato chips. After an argument with her mother, she doesn't hit the 24-hour diner across the street from her apartment. Instead, she opens the freezer and grabs a peanut butter cup. Clearly, emotional eating isn't about gourmet food or fine dining. It's about convenience and immediacy. It's about grabbing whatever's in sight or within reach.

IS BOREDOM PLAYING HAVOC
WITH YOUR WAISTLINE?

"Boredom eaters" are different. Unlike run-of-the-mill mood eaters, boredom eaters don't discriminate: the act of eating is more important than what they eat. Most mood eaters seek out favorite snacks. Boredom eaters aren't so choosy. They're looking to fill time and will munch anything within arm's reach.

Unstructured time is the enemy of boredom eaters. One reason most diets are successful in the short term is that they give clear structure to people who are often out of control with food. The most obvious characteristic of boredom eating is that it's totally devoid of structure. I have a client who spent three weeks at home recovering from lower back surgery. After 20 games of Scrabble, 50 Sex and the City reruns, 40 hours on Facebook and Twitter, and $2,000 worth of online shopping for things she didn't need, my client found herself wandering idly over to the refrigerator. Pulling open two large gleaming steel doors, she would gaze vaguely into her refrigerator's brightly lit, inviting interior, waiting for inspiration to strike. That's boredom eating. If hunger had been the issue, she would have pulled the trigger much sooner.

When it comes to boredom eating, structure is the cure. Plan a non-eating activity. Gardening, reading, cleaning, talking on the phone, or texting your friend—nearly any food-free activity is a better use of your time than swan-diving into a bag of potato chips. Accomplishing something that's personally rewarding is an instant cure for boredom.

Of course, even the most disciplined, scheduled person is going to end up with free time on his or her hands, and as we all know, "the devil finds work for idle hands." I tell many clients who struggle with boredom eating to keep a supply of healthy, low-calorie snacks around the house, such as crudité (minus the high-calorie dipping sauce), low-calorie, single-serving bags of popcorn (provided it's not a bad boyfriend), or high-fiber, low-calorie crackers such as GG Bran Crispbread or a Ryvita Rye & Oat High-Fiber Bran Cracker or Crispbread. Avoid small, high-calorie finger foods such as chips or brownies and similar snacks for which ease and convenience are the main selling points. As well, never make grocery shopping, cooking, or baking your boredom-conquering activity. Even cleaning the kitchen might prove too tempting for some.

We all do the same things every day. The idea is not necessarily to change what we're doing but to look at things in a different way. As Marcel Proust said, "The real voyage of discovery consists not in seeking new landscapes but in having new eyes." Find a new view. Remember that if boredom turns into boredom eating, you could end up bored to death.

Why Don't We Crave Apples?

HAVE YOU NOTICED THAT EMOTIONAL EATING ALMOST NEVER IN-volves apples, carrots, or a cup of nonfat yogurt? When was the last time you binged on a bowl of broccoli or bag of snow peas? After another aggravating afternoon with your in-laws, why don't you indulge in a Jell-O cup or a handful of grapes? The intense, "need something right now" feeling—better known as a craving—sends us sprinting to the fattiest, sweetest, and most calorie-rich treat we can get our hands on. Why?

Much of the answer may lie in our evolutionary history. Scientists suspect that we're genetically predisposed to grab the most caloric foods we can find. At the dawn of human history, food was often in short supply. It makes sense that we'd possess some sort of internal mechanism that would drive us to consume the most calories possible. Turns out, our ancestors' brains probably responded to the sudden calorie upsurge resulting from a hearty meal by releasing dopamine and serotonin, the "feel-good" neurotransmitters that release "feel-good" chemicals. This surge of hormones—prompted directly by sugary, high-fat, high-caloric foods—is associated with happiness, pleasure, and contentment. These foods are so powerful that their impact on the brain's reward pathway is much the same as the impact of drug abuse. This explains why celery sticks are rarely the first choice after a job loss, a financial problem, or a dustup with your mother-in-law. Our minds are still compensating for a perceived lack of resources, even though we're awash in McDonald's, Wendy's, Domino's, and Krispy Kreme. And it doesn't take much to trigger the "feast or famine" mindset. Any sort of emotional trauma—real or imagined—is enough to send most of us in the direction of the nearest bag of Fritos.

Are We Wired to Eat This Way?

It's no stretch to say that incentives motivate perfor-mance. The promise of a year-end bonus can motivate an employee to work harder. She wants to do a bang-up job, but certainly the promise of cold hard cash is the driving force here. On the other hand, a man who helps his brother-in-law install a new flat-screen TV in his den is rewarded with the feeling that he's doing something nice for a family member. The latter is an example of a natural reward that results from being altruistic. Helping out is a reward in and of itself because it feels good. Contrast that with the employee who's busting her hump for a sizable year-end bonus. The work-for-bonus incentive system is an example of an artificial reward.

The artificially rewarding feelings we derive from food trump any sort of natural reward, something scholars are only just learning. In a study presented at a meeting of the prestigious Society for the Study of Ingestive Behavior (SSIB)—the foremost organization for research into all aspects of eating and drinking behavior—researchers found that ghrelin, the hormone that stimulates feeding, is closely linked to dopamine, the feel-good neurotransmitter, within the striatum, a critical component of the brain's reward system.

In the study, scientists measured dopamine levels in real time while rats ate sugar, a highly rewarding and thus addictive food. Administering ghrelin to rats while they ate sugar increased peak dopamine spikes within the striatum, whereas administering a drug that blocks ghrelin's action significantly reduced dopamine levels during sugar intake. Dr. Mitch Roitman, the author of the study, told *Science News Daily* that "the modulation of brain dopamine reward signals by a gut hormone that regulates appetite strongly supports this interaction as a way to direct the organism's behavior towards further intake, perhaps by making food more rewarding."

Of course, none of this information matters to mood eaters. They don't need scientific studies to know about the rewarding effects of sweet, creamy, sugary, salty, and crunchy foods. For most of them, the reward from a doughnut, cupcake, or chocolate bar blows away helping a little old lady across the street and explains why they opt for a handful of Oreo cookies over a cup of fresh-cut bell peppers. Oreos act on the brain's reward pathway—the mesolimbic dopamine system—in much the same way drugs do. So while it's great to have your spouse or partner rub your shoulders after a long hard day, to most mood eaters a shoulder massage places a distant second to a pint of Häagen-Dazs mint chocolate chip ice cream.

Even happy feelings can trigger mood eating. My client Linda decided to go back to work after her youngest child entered elementary school. Within an hour of learning that she'd found a job, Linda was arm-deep in a bag of Doritos. As Brian Wansink, Ph.D., director of the Food and Brand Lab at Cornell University, points out, "Comfort foods are often wrongly associated with negative moods, and indeed, people often consume them when they're down or depressed, but interestingly enough, comfort foods are also consumed to maintain good moods." What Dr. Wansink is saying is that any shift in our feeling equilibrium—good or bad— is uncomfortable. We're looking to restore balance so we turn to food, even if we're happy. Of course, you're not going to be happy if you gain 30 pounds and go up three sizes.

ANXIOUS OR HUNGRY?
HOW TO TELL THE DIFFERENCE

We now know that food "feeds" our feelings as well as our stomachs. But how can you tell which is which? Here are some basic differences between physical and emotional hunger:

1. Emotional hunger comes on suddenly; physical hunger is gradual.

2. Mood eating is specific. Most mood eaters are looking to quickly fill a need, so high-fat, high-carb finger foods like potato chips, bite-size cookies, and crackers are often the first option. Mood eaters aren't interested in seeking variety, sitting down to a fancy gourmet meal, or nourishing their bodies.

3. Emotional eaters keep chowing down even when they're full. If you're eating because you're hungry, you're more likely to stop when you feel full.

4. Emotional eaters have survivor's guilt. They always feel horrible, particularly after a binge. People who eat when they're hungry don't carry the same burden.

5. Mood eaters resemble animals scavenging over a carcass. They eat as quickly as possible. The faster the food goes down, the quicker they find relief for their uncomfortable emotions or feelings. On the other hand, I think most people find it a lot more pleasurable to slow down the pace at mealtime. After all, who wants to rush through dinner at a fine restaurant? I don't know a single mood eater who takes time to savor the taste, presentation, and preparation of food.

6. Mood eating is like watching pornography. It's typically done in isolation. When was the last time you binged on cookie dough in front of your colleagues or tore through a plate of French fries in front of a guy you were trying to impress? There are few greater pleasures in life than enjoying a celebratory meal with family or friends.

Where Emotional Eating Comes From, and How to Stop It

I CAN TALK TO YOU UNTIL I'M IN BLUE IN THE FACE ABOUT THE TOLL that emotional eating takes on your body. But most dieters care more about fitting into their skinny jeans. The call to health is often secondary to the call to look amazing.

Either way, the path is the same, even if the priorities are not. Emotional overeating is a leading cause of weight gain, and addressing the root cause is critical. Awareness is the first step to overcoming emotional eating. It may seem obvious, but many mood eaters don't even recognize that they're doing it! In all likelihood, this is a behavior that started in childhood and has been reinforced over time. Every day children are admonished to "clean their plates." Parents use food as a reward, treat, or goodie. As adults, many of us never break free of this early life conditioning. We eat everything on our plates. We eat to feel good, and we eat to feel better. We eat to reward ourselves after a hard day at work.

A cookie, candy bar, or bag of pretzels may very well have been the perfect reward for a physically active seven-year-old who never struggled with her weight. But It Girls know that part of growing up in the world of food is to let go of the emotional programming and cultural conditioning of your childhood. A cookie, Hershey bar, or other bad boyfriend won't improve a lousy day, pay off your debt, or get your husband to help you around the house.

If you've always used comfort food to push away uncomfortable feelings, then you might find that reality—learning how to deal with feelings without the aid of food—is hard. But we have to start somewhere, and building emotional skills is a good place to start. Take a Mr. Spock approach to emotional eating. Mr. Spock is the most logical of the crew on *Star Trek*. Though taking the emotion out of emotional eating is easier said than done, the Skinny Jeans Diet will help you become more logical in the way you think about food.

The Deprivation-Obsession Connection

WANT TO KNOW THE NUMBER-ONE REASON PEOPLE FAIL ON A DIET? They feel like they're missing out. Deprivation, especially when it comes to food, is a powerful experience. Why do millions of people cheat on their spouses? Experts will tell you that something is missing from their lives. An affair is a last-ditch attempt to fill a void. Love, sex, or attention—they're searching for something they're just not getting at home. Dieters stray for the same reason: they feel deprived.

No one—dieters least of all—wants to be on the outside looking in. Imagine waiting all year for your mother's Thanksgiving dinner and limiting yourself to celery sticks, undressed salad, and a few slices of dry turkey while everyone around you indulges in sweet potatoes, stuffing, cranberry sauce, and pumpkin pie. Hello? It's Thanksgiving. You wouldn't head to the Barney's semiannual warehouse sale to buy a pair of shoelaces or a T-shirt, would you? I don't think so. I'll take five skirts, four blouses, three dresses, and a second helping of everything, please! Imagine spending six months eating rabbit food just so you can finally fit into that new $300 bikini. According to psychologists, the moment you banish a food, it paradoxically builds up a "craving life" of its own that increases in momentum as the deprivation deepens.

Following that train of thought, depriving yourself of a food you want all but guarantees that you're going to overeat that very item. Think back to your childhood. Do you remember how you felt when your parents told you that you couldn't have something? Didn't that make you want it that much more? It's the power of the forbidden fruit.

Take lip gloss, for example. Want to create a crazy craving for lip gloss? Deprive yourself of it for a week or two. You can wear mascara, blush, eye shadow, eyeliner, and perfume, but not lip gloss. Guess what you'll be craving in about 15 minutes?

Telling yourself you can't have something intensifies its appeal and allure. This is especially the case when it comes to food. According to cutting-edge research from the University of Toronto, making treats—even the very naughtiest bad boyfriends—totally off limits could easily undo your weight loss efforts. In one study, female dieters who were deprived of chocolate for a week had more intense cravings than those without any food restrictions, and they consumed two times more chocolate than usual when they were finally permitted to eat it. "When you cut something out of your diet, you're more likely to overeat that very thing when you do encounter it," said Janet Polivy, Ph.D., the study's lead author. When you rigidly limit the amount or types of food you are allowed to eat, you're usually setting yourself up to crave larger quantities of that very food.

If you find yourself plowing through a bag of pretzels or munching uncontrollably on M&Ms, it could be because something is missing from your life. You may be scared and disgusted by your own behavior, but you don't know how to stop. What do you do then? Like most dieters, you look for a measure of control: you restrict yourself even more and end up feeling more deprived in the process. You may stop going out, break plans, and focus all your energy on your restrictive diet. This in turn can lead to a feeling of powerlessness and inertia. You feel stuck emotionally. And what do emotional eaters who feel stuck emotionally do? They eat!

If deprivation leads to overeating, weight gain, and feeling out of control with food, what's the solution? How do you end the destructive pattern of deprivation and weight gain?

The answer is to have "good guy" alternatives on hand so you never feel deprived. Today there's probably a delicious, low-calorie alternative for nearly every bad boy food you love. This should come as welcome news to dieters. After all, who wants to go to a birthday bash or engagement party and stare longingly at a piece of shrimp and a glass of seltzer while everyone else eats to their heart's content? Talk about buzz kill! As dieters, it's a strategy—not just a preference—to make ourselves part of the party. So go to that party—but this time, arm yourself with winning strategies. Don't worry: they'll fit into the pocket of your skinny jeans.

Tips and Tricks to End the Cycle of Emotional Eating

1. **Stop bringing those naughty men home.** This is the number-one strategy to end emotional eating. Don't bring nibble-size bad boyfriends into the house! You can't eat what's not there. Remember, mood eaters want convenience. They're interested in foods that can be popped into their mouths quickly and easily; they're not going to sit down to a fancy meal. Protecting your home environment is the first step to putting an end to emotional eating.

2. **Don't go hungry.** You're less likely to reach for bad boyfriends and other nibble foods if you feel full. Along with your regular meals, pencil in two or three snacks of no more than 150 calories each. Many dieters find that light midmorning and midafternoon snacks help stave off hunger. Just make sure your choice of snack isn't a bad

boyfriend. And don't worry if you feel the need to have one of these snacks late at night. Calories consumed after dark are no more detrimental to your weight than those eaten during the day. Calories are calories. It doesn't matter what time you eat them. What matters is the number of calories you consume!

3. **Keep an emergency "first-aid food kit" with you at all times.** A client once told me that whenever she goes out, she always brings a makeup kit, even if it's just for a quick run to the grocery store. This might seem a little obsessive, but as she says, "You never know who you might run into." Similarly, mood eaters should never go anywhere without a first-aid food kit. This can be an insulated bag or cooler filled with meals and snacks that you plan on eating that day. These meals and snacks shouldn't vary too much. Although it may seem boring to eat the same thing every day, studies show that variety stimulates consumption, whereas people who have fewer food choices lose more weight. With an emergency food kit, you'll never again find yourself flying by the seat of your pants.

4. **Find an alternative.** It may seem obvious, but if emotional eating causes you to reach for a cookie or candy bar, consider a great-tasting, low-calorie alternative. If a setback at work triggers chocolate cravings, you don't necessarily have to give up your favorite food, provided it's not a really bad boyfriend. Instead, save your needless aggravation and

hundreds of calories with one of Chocolite's great-tasting, low-calorie alternatives. At 35 to 100 calories, these moist, chewy, and delicious chocolate bars are packed with fiber and protein, which promote satiety and help you feel full longer.

5. **Distract yourself away from food.** Whether it's walking, listening to music, cleaning, phoning, or Skyping, any non-eating activity can divert your attention when emotional hunger strikes.

6. **It's not the end of the world.** Every dieter who has ever lived has fallen off the wagon. Don't make too much of your mistakes. Strive for progress, not perfection. If you polish off two or three cupcakes after a dustup with your hubby, let it go. Balance out your latest binge with a generous helping of vegetables or high-fiber, low-calorie fruit, such as an apple, with your next meal or snack.

7. **Keep a food diary.** Every girl needs a little black book. It Girls know that a food record is vital to staying organized and on top of their game. You can't undo what you've done, but you can certainly change your perspective on it. If you blow it one day, consider why that happened. Many women find that keeping a record of their daily food intake or writing down a detailed food plan helps them stay on track, whether they're trying to lose weight or maintain their weight and activity levels.

8. **Freshen your breath.** I don't have any studies to prove it, but I've found that brushing your teeth, using a breath strip, or popping a strong mint or some chewing gum blocks cravings and makes food less appetizing, all while making you a lot more kissable. You can also try eating grapefruit, some parsley, or an orange, all of which have a similarly cleansing effect as they help rid your mouth and mind of the taste of the bad boyfriend foods that trigger emotional eating.

9. **Close the kitchen.** Your kitchen isn't a 24-hour diner. Set a time when you're going to clean up, turn off the lights, and announce that the kitchen is closed for business. I have a client who shuts down her kitchen every night at 8:00 P.M. without fail. If her husband happens to come home late from work and hasn't eaten dinner, he knows he has to pick up his own dinner. My client tells him, "Hi, honey, you are on your own." Remember, a lot of mood eating takes place at night, so the earlier you do this the skinnier you're going to be.

10. **Spend quality time in a nonfood room.** I have a client who likes to work late at her kitchen table. Hello? This is no different from a recovering addict killing time in a crack den. Even the most spartan kitchen is full of cues that trigger overeating. Have you ever heard of a refrigerator? Remember that when it comes to mood eating, convenience and availability are key. If food is in sight and within arm's reach, you're going to pounce. In

one experiment, chocolate candies were put in plain view on office workers' desks. On average, the workers ate nine pieces each per day and often lost track of how many they'd eaten. Conversely, when the chocolate was out of sight and at least six feet from their desks, the workers averaged just four. Mood eaters are even lazy about their overeating! If you need to work, why not work in the living room or den? If possible, avoid the kitchen except for mealtime. I have one client who keeps a toddler gate on the entrance to her kitchen during nonmeal times even though her children are grown and out of the house. The gate is a reminder to steer clear, especially when the urge to binge strikes. Good fences make good neighbors, not to mention thin waists!

Build an Imaginary Shield

THERE ARE ROUGHLY 75 MILLION ACTIVE DIETERS IN THIS COUNtry. If you were to take a survey of them, nearly all would tell you a tale of woe about emotional eating.

Say your husband comes home from work and starts venting about his lousy day. In no time flat he's talking about the weak economy and impending layoffs at his company and telling you, "No new shoes for a month." When this happens at my house, I'm always tempted to reach for the cookie dough. Fortunately, I've developed an effective trick for controlling my reactions.

I picture an imaginary shield around me that allows me to hear and acknowledge what my husband is saying. Yet this amazing, imaginary shield bounces away all the negative stuff, so that I don't absorb and internalize any of it. If I absorbed it, it could drive me straight to the kids' junk food drawer and keep me up all night searching for a pair of pants to zip over my new "Oreo bump" the next day. The imaginary shield is my way of coping with worry and fear, as well as my husband's meshugah. It helps me to stay in the here and now so that I can remain calm, practice positive self-talk, and refrain from drowning my worries with food. Miraculously, staying calm makes me feel calm, which lessens my need to eat.

You can't control everything in life. You can't control your circumstances. You can't even control your efforts. But you can always control your reactions. One such reaction is to make the adult choice not to run to food when you're feeling stressed, anxious, or angry. This isn't always easy—if it was, you wouldn't be reading this book—but with the right skills it can be done. Building your own imaginary shield is a great place to begin.

Breaking Free

JUST A SHORT 15 YEARS AGO, I BROKE THE NASTY CYCLE OF BINGE-eating and started living thin. Still, in my heart of hearts, I'm a mood eater and always will be. When I'm anxious, I eat. I did this when I was tipping the scales at 190, and I still feel the urge to do it now at a healthy 120. To this day words of disapproval from my husband or mother or an impending deadline at work send me straight to food. The only difference is that I'm more careful about what I binge on. My binges are shorter, and I have an easier time talking myself down from the ledge. Instead of seeking shelter in a bag of Doritos or snuggling up alongside a Pillsbury cookie dough log, I created a list of 20 to 25 "comfort" foods that won't wreck my life or waistline. My favorites are baby carrots with gobs of honey mustard, rice cakes with a wedge of

Laughing Cow Light Cheese (and more honey mustard), or a single-serving bag of lightly salted, unbuttered popcorn. Elimination may not be realistic, but replacement is.

Since overeating is a disease of thinking, changing the thoughts and behaviors that trigger emotional eating can help. Cognitive behavioral therapy is a short-term approach that encourages the positive behaviors that will help you combat the thoughts that trigger mood eating. It's surprisingly effective. Studies have shown that lifestyle changes encourage greater weight loss when paired with cognitive behavioral therapy. First, you change your thoughts. Then you alter your feelings. Finally, you change your actions. It's a perfect one-two-three punch!

Even on those rare occasions when I do fall off the wagon, I feel secure since my home environment is protected. I don't shovel fatty, sugary, high-calorie foods into my mouth because I've banished them from my house. (Save for the kids' junk food drawer, which I keep under lock and key. When the kids want a snack, I usually ask my husband, who doesn't have a food problem, to open it for them.) My downside—and more important, backside—is protected.

No matter why or what you're eating, the outcome is always the same with emotional eating. You can be overwhelmed and thin, or overwhelmed and fat. The thing to do is to recognize when you're overwhelmed and learn some behavioral techniques to help you when the urge to eat hits. Below are some favorite strategies my clients have shared over the years.

1. Read an absorbing book
2. Rent or go to a movie
3. Call a friend
4. Clean out your closet

5. Buy yourself a small, nonfood present

6. Get a facial or massage

7. Buy yourself flowers

8. Read a self-help book

9. Do a puzzle or Sudoku

10. Surf the Internet

11. Take a nap

12. Write in a journal

13. Get some new makeup or a haircut

14. Get together with a friend

15. Play with your kids

16. Exercise

17. Garden or start a household project

18. Paint your nails

19. Get professional counseling

20. Join a support group

Along with these strategies, It Girls follow five simple rules that all but ensure that they never fall into the mood eating trap.

1. **Do something nice for yourself.** When their mood eating urge hits, I encourage clients to ask themselves, "What can I do right now to make myself feel better?" My client Debra commutes daily to New York City, works 10-hour days, and then comes home to the usual evening routine of kids and household chores. For years she'd walk through the door and make a beeline for the fridge. It was the only path she seemed to know into her house. Often she'd start eating with her coat still on. After working on strategies

for relaxing without food, Debra discovered that she loves getting into her sleep socks and loungewear when she comes home from work. The clothes are warm, cozy, soft, and soothing ("even better than food," she would say).

If you're feeling lonely, how about calling a friend? If you're bored, pick up a good book or watch a favorite movie. If you're exhausted, then turn in earlier. If you're feeling stressed, then why not take a walk? If you're feeling down, buy yourself flowers. I think you get the picture. There are lots of healthy, nonfood distractions out there. Find one that works for you.

2. **Don't shop when you're hungry.** Do you want to have a hard time sticking with your Skinny Jeans Diet grocery list? Try grocery shopping on an empty stomach. In a study presented at the 2011 conference of the Society for the Study of Ingestive Behavior, participants were injected with either ghrelin, a hormone that increases hunger, or a saline solution, then asked to bid on both edible treats and nonfood items. Ghrelin increased what participants were willing to pay for food, but decreased what they were willing to pay for everything else. In other words, the brain's reward system was more responsive to the food than to other goodies—even a fancy designer handbag! Ghrelin biased the brain toward craving calories! This makes perfect sense since, if you're starving, nothing will distract you on the way to the nearest food source. Bottom line: don't think of loading up your shopping cart under the influence of an underfed appetite.

3. **Beware of flashy packages.** Bright colors and patterns in nature often mean danger. In the world of food, bright colors and patterns amount to the same thing. As we learned in the bad boyfriends chapter, food manufacturers spend billions each year on product placement, aesthetics, and advertising to get you to buy, even those things you don't want or need. Have you ever wondered why Cheetos come in a flashy orange bag? Because no one would eat them if they were in a plain black one.

4. **Have a plan, but keep it flexible.** "Blessed are the hearts that can bend; they shall never be broken," said Albert Camus. Planning is critical to structuring and organizing your food environment. But you have to be flexible. Some girls may feel their day is wrecked if they have to vary their eating plan because their schedule changes or their favorite foods are unavailable. But the elite 3 percent understand that being flexible is part of living thin. If an emergency meeting comes up at work and you don't have time for your afternoon snack, make sure you grab an eight-ounce cup of cold water, which studies show can make you feel full and stave off hunger. And be sure to grab your snack as soon as the meeting ends (having your emergency food kit on hand can really help). It may take a little extra work, but it will keep you on track. In addition, there are multiple apps, many of them free, from sites like Sparkpeople and Calorie King that can help organize your food day.

5. **Be conceited.** Jot down one compliment each day in your food diary. It doesn't have to come from someone else. It can be something you make up. And make it as specific as possible: "My hair looks like Jennifer Lopez's today," or "I was so patient this morning getting the kids off to school." Finding something nice to say about yourself helps build self-esteem and confidence. It will help you feel better, which in turn will motivate you to make better food decisions.

Keeping It All in Perspective

THIN OR FAT, FOR MOST GIRLS FOOD IS ONE OF LIFE'S GREAT PLEA-sures. For emotional eaters, the problem really isn't the food; it's one of perspective.

Emotional eaters don't view food as a source of nourishment or pleasure but as a vehicle for protecting themselves from painful feelings and emotions. For mood eaters, what they put in their mouths has nothing to do with what they eat and everything to do with how they feel. Self-care is noticeably absent, though it may appear otherwise to girls who are caught in the web of emotional food choices.

Girls who have successfully broken the torrid pattern of emotional eating don't just "get a grip" or "talk themselves out of it." Food psychology is complex. Unraveling our ingrained habits, especially those related to food, is a process of exploration and self-discovery, awareness building, and self-mastery.

The It Girls know that there's no cause for despair, even for those who have spent a lifetime caught in the throes of mood eating. There's light at the end of the tunnel. A positive outlook on life, a healthy attitude toward yourself, and overall optimism have a direct impact on your ability to break free of mood eating. You can change the feelings of boredom, depression, low self-esteem, and loneliness that plague you into new, empowering actions without the help of chocolate chip cookies or a bag of potato chips.

If you're still worried, don't be—you can learn new thinking skills and take positive action steps. Below is a list of my favorites.

1. **Wait it out.** Wait 10 minutes. Distract yourself. Chances are, the urge to eat will ease.
2. **Write it out.** Remember your first diary when you were 12 years old? Pick one up again and write down your foods and moods. It made you feel better then, and it will make you thinner now! Address your feelings head-on.
3. **Talk it out.** Talk to someone who can calm and support you. Talking it out can give you clarity on what the issue is.
4. **Sweat it out.** Though its contribution to weight loss is minimal, any physical activity provides a great emotional release.
5. **Think it out.** Positive thinking can help you walk yourself off of the bad boyfriend ledge. Tell yourself, *I've been doing so well. Are those few cookies really worth a few months of feeling out of control and miserable?*

A Light at the Back of the Fridge

YOUR LIFE WON'T ALWAYS BE GREAT. IN FACT, IT'S GOING TO SUCK sometimes. "To live is to suffer," said Gautama Buddha. Uncomfortable emotions, vexing problems, and untenable situations are a part of the human condition—get used to them. They'll be there whether you're living on carrot sticks and kale or drowning your sorrows in a vat of Oreos. You can handle life's challenges fat or you can handle them thin. I've done both, and I can say confidently that thin is better. You run your household, small business, and children's schedules. Food shouldn't get in the way of all you need to do. It's the twenty-first century. How long are you going to let a cookie be your boss, judge, savior, or executioner?

CHAPTER 5

Cravings

YOU'RE IN THE SUPERMARKET WHEN HE CATCHES YOUR eye—the gorgeous young buck you used to date. It's been years but feels like only yesterday that you were hot and heavy. And damn does he look good. He runs those rugged hands through that thick mane of curly black hair. Beads of perspiration gather on your brow; you feel like you're about to pass out. That simple gesture causes a sinking feeling in the pit of your stomach. Now you're reminiscing. *He was the best thing that ever happened to me. How did it go so wrong?* At that moment, all the hurt feelings, broken promises, bad habits, passes at other women, and glib comments about your mother seem like a distant memory. What harm could there be in "accidentally" bumping into him as he's checking out the sweet potatoes? Slowly you make your way over, tap him on the shoulder, and give him a coy smile.

Much to your amazement and delight, he's thrilled to see you. Before long, you're chatting online, texting, talking on the phone, meeting for coffee, and hooking up for wild sex.

It's an unwritten rule that you're supposed to give yourself half the length of time that your relationship lasted to get over it. But this rule ignores the insidiousness of the ex-bad boyfriend life cycle. The sex, the "over it but not really over it" drama, the endless boxes of tissues, and the anguished late-night phone calls to your girlfriends keep you stuck in a never-ending cycle of misery and self-loathing.

If this is your pattern, I have three words for you: *Turn back now!* Remember, you broke up for a reason. It's called a breakup because it's broken.

Seeing an ex-bad boyfriend can be exhilarating and unnerving— much like encountering a rich, fattening food you once loved but, after years of heartache and increasingly larger pant sizes, finally found the courage to quit. Just as hooking up with your ex can rekindle the toxic relationship cycle, going back to a bad boyfriend food can quickly turn a harmless little food craving into an all-out feeding frenzy.

We're usually young and impressionable the first time we fall head over heels, and the result is a lasting physical and chemical imprint. Reigniting these emotional memories reignites our feelings, only they're stronger and even more resilient this time around. The same holds true for food cravings. Studies have shown that people have cravings memories. Literally, cravings start in your head, not your belly. Simply thinking about food or even talking about it can unleash urges, and those urges always seem to be for our bad boyfriends.

Some girls try going cold turkey, thinking they can turn off the cravings faucet with a strict, no-contact policy. Hello? Remember the brief supermarket encounter with the ex? How'd that turn out? You were back in the saddle in no time flat. Telling yourself that your bad boyfriend is off limits only increases your cravings for him. He's the proverbial forbidden fruit. (It's too bad our bad boyfriend foods aren't actually fruit. We wouldn't have so many problems swearing them off.)

I have a client who recently swore off gummy candies. While this seemed like a sound idea, within a week she was fantasizing and obsessing about Sour Patch Kids. A study by researchers at the University of Chicago found that abstinence increases cravings for food and that food cues further increased cravings even after a period of abstinence. How else to explain why the ex can still drive you nuts even though he's been out of the picture for years? Rigidly limiting the quantities and kinds of food you're allowed to eat makes you crave more of that very food, and you set yourself up to fail.

Here's the other thing you need to know about cravings: talk is cheap. Even the most determined girls are hard-pressed to talk themselves out of cravings. Dieters who try to squash or eat around a craving wind up consuming about 40 percent more calories. The cravings memory is strong, as our man Mr. Proust observed. So what's a girl to do when her past calls?

Like getting over a bad ex, there are some hard and fast dos and don'ts for conquering a food craving.

> **Do remember why you broke up.** Though your natural impulse might be to get back together, never forget why your relationship went down the toilet in the first place. So the next time you bump into a handsome bucket of movie theater popcorn, stop and think about how your encounter left you feeling bloated, fat, and pissed off. Think: *Do I really want to get myself in that situation again?*

Don't hook up. Seeing your ex unexpectedly is like seeing the Good Humor truck and suddenly wanting ice cream. Hooking up is a bad idea because it prolongs the drama and makes the inevitable separation that much harder.

Do plan for run-ins. If you know that bumping into your ex may throw you for a loop, try to avoid being in places where you know he may turn up, such as the bakery. Still, you never know who you're going to run into, so make a plan in case you encounter that gorgeous hunk of cream-filled cake at your son's school play. At pastry-filled school functions, some of my clients make a beeline for the ladies' room, while others distract themselves by talking to other moms. Just be careful not to nibble. Remember that your ex is a compulsion, and when did you ever have just a little of a compulsion?

Do think positive. Remember how it feels to be confident, happy, and hot in your new skinny jeans.

Bad boyfriend foods come in all flavors, shapes, and sizes. My client Bonnie has been trying to kick a chocolate-covered-everything habit for years. Pretzels, nuts, cookies, candy, graham crackers, marshmallows—if it comes with chocolate, Bonnie will abuse it. On top of that, Bonnie is a mood eater, and few foods are more dangerous for mood eaters than chocolate. Even the high-fiber chocolate-bar substitute I gave Bonnie triggered cravings and out-of-control eating. She needed a chocolate alternative with different textures that she didn't normally seek out or encounter in her day-to-day life. I recommended that Bonnie try individual cups of fat-free chocolate mousse, Jell-O pudding, a Healthy Choice Fudge Bar, or a low-calorie chocolate shake, such as Alba 70.

I have another client who made a habit of abusing fruit pie. It wasn't uncommon for her to devour an entire pie in a single sitting. I gave her my recipe for baked apples (see page 274), which weighs in at one-third of the calories and wasn't something she was likely to abuse. (Who abuses apples?) You can even skip the food option and go for Extra Dessert Delights Sugar-Free Gum, which incidentally comes in apple pie flavor. If you love mashed potatoes, try my Mock Mashed Potatoes (see page 209), which has great taste and texture for half the calories. The main idea is to trick your taste buds into being satisfied with a lighter way of eating and enjoying the foods that work for you and not against you.

The Power of Hedonic Hunger

HAVE YOU EVER GIVEN IN TO A GORGEOUS SLAB OF CHOCOLATE cake or a freshly baked baguette, not because you were hungry, but because you wanted it? This is known as "hedonic hunger," and it's basically the immediate need for food that brings pleasure. It helps explain why you keep giving in to those foods you keep swearing off.

Recently, a group of Italian scientists discovered that when we eat for pleasure rather than hunger, a reward chemical known as 2-AG and the hunger hormone ghrelin are significantly activated, which leads us to desire food based on how it tastes rather than as an energy source. Clearly, hedonic hunger stimulates overeating, and it's especially dangerous in an environment where our bad boyfriend foods are present.

Here's the other problem with hedonic hunger. It's not satisfying. Like any form of immediate gratification, the sensation passes quickly and we have to keep doing it again and again to achieve the same result. It's really no different than drugs, sex, gambling, or shopping—anything that creates a sensation that dissipates quickly.

My client Beth has been fighting a losing battle with tortilla chips for years. She goes to every party and social event determined not to let this bad boy get the best of her. She can usually make it through without too much damage. But the mental obsession—images of those crispy, salty chips dancing in her head—lingers. She thinks about the chips while washing her face and brushing her teeth. Like clockwork, Beth finds herself downstairs in her dark kitchen, elbow deep in the bag of "healthy" veggie chips. In an instant, she's polished off most of the 1,300-calorie bag. Now you see why many so-called healthy foods are anything but. Beth would have been better off with a single-serving bag of Way Better Snacks Simply Sunny Multi-Grain Tortilla Chips for just 137 calories.

The Big Tease

ANOTHER DEFINING CHARACTERISTIC OF THE FOODS WE CRAVE IS that they're calorie-dense: they contain mega-calories relative to their small portion size. Dieters by nature are volume eaters. And calorie-dense foods seldom give us a bang for our buck. Small portion sizes leave most people feeling unsatisfied or deprived. Let's not forget as well that the most calorie-dense foods are almost invariably our bad boyfriends.

A recent Tufts University study confirmed that while almost all people have cravings, only some give in to their must-haves, albeit less often or with a close runner-up. They know that completely denying cravings can lead to bingeing later on. They accept that cravings are a normal part of life that has to be dealt with.

But giving in to temptation is by no means a black-and-white choice. Sometimes ladies indulge their cravings, but in controlled portions. Other gals find that even a taste reignites their inner Proust and that it's better not to get involved at all.

Should You Stray?

IMAGINE TELLING YOUR SIGNIFICANT OTHER THAT ONE DAY A week you need a little roll in the hay with someone else. Well, that's exactly what millions of otherwise faithful dieters do: one day a week they cheat on their eating plan and eat anything they want—and lots of it.

But is a cheat day a bad thing? While your spouse might not take kindly to your hooking up with some hot dude, many experts argue, and studies bear out, that dieters should incorporate cheat days into their eating plan, since too much deprivation can increase cravings, causing you to fall off the wagon.

Another reason for cheating, say the experts, is that radically spiking your calorie intake effectively resets the thyroid gland, which controls your metabolism, and stops the deceleration of your fat loss. Remember how thrilled you were to watch the pounds drop off and the dress size shrink? When you first start dieting, weight loss is often dramatic. But in no time the losses decrease. A cheat day may help trigger your body's "I just started dieting" response.

Here's one thing the experts are missing, however. For most dieters, cheat days involve a naughty encounter with a bad boyfriend. For some ladies, this is perfectly fine. After a quick hook-up, they happily move on their way. For the majority of skinny gals, however, starting up with their bad boyfriend foods reignites cravings and triggers overeating. So if you decide to stray, be careful that your cheat day doesn't turn into a lifetime of infidelity.

Clients often ask me: how do you control a cheat day? The one hard and fast rule I have is that if you're going to stray, don't cheat with a guy who's going to cause you to want to leave your family. In other words, don't cheat with a food that's going to reactivate a lifetime of cravings.

Every two weeks I allow myself a cheat day. My husband and I go out to a nice restaurant. I'll enjoy the bread basket, perhaps some pasta, and I may even have a few French fries. I can do this because I can enjoy these foods without overeating them. Under no circumstances, however, do I allow myself dessert. I simply can't control myself around sweet baked goods. Years ago, I made an adult decision that I needed to cut them out of my life. If the food you're cheating with is a food you've never been able to control yourself around, you have to ask yourself, *Am I going to change?* For me, the writing was on the wall. If you make an honest assessment, you'll see that the writing is on the wall for you as well.

CRAVE WITH CONVICTION

If you're going to give in to a craving, do it with gusto. Go ahead and eat that (one) candy, provided it's not a choice that's going to cause you to lose control and it's something you really want. If you love Twix bars, then go to a convenience store, buy a single Twix bar, and savor every bite. Don't buy a different candy bar because it's on sale. (Remember, when dieters eat "around" a craving, they eat 40 percent more.) Have your favorite, make sure it's portion-controlled (don't buy an entire bag of Twix Mini Bars, telling yourself you'll have just one or two and the rest are for the kids!), and eat it with passion. The key is to indulge only on occasion and be truly satisfied.

Are We Programmed to Pig Out?

HOW MANY TIMES HAVE YOU HEARD YOUR BFF TALK ABOUT HER addiction to cookies, candy, or French fries? After hearing another horror story about a ruined figure at the hand of a slice of chocolate cake or a scoop of cookie dough ice cream, you may even wonder if you suffer from that problem yourself. In fact, we're all wired to get a chemical rush from calorie-rich treats. As Nora Volkow, director of the National Institute on Drug Abuse and an expert on the science of addiction, points out, "We're programmed to pig out on calories."

According to Susan Roberts, Ph.D., professor of nutrition and psychology at Tufts University in Boston, "When you bite into something delicious, like your favorite junk food, your brain releases dopamine, the same 'reward chemical' that kicks in during sex and drug use, just in a smaller amount."

How do you beat back your brain's powerful neurochemical response? Make sure you have your personal good guy food on hand and schedule it into your daily food plan. I've found that clients who know they'll be eating something they enjoy have fewer cravings and are less likely to feel deprived. I tell clients that every afternoon and evening they need to schedule a 100- to 200-calorie snack, which many find makes it easier to resist a conference room full of pastries at four in the afternoon.

The Diet Witching Hour

SPEAKING OF THE AFTERNOON HOURS, HOW MANY TIMES HAVE YOU fallen prey to the late-afternoon munchies? Late-afternoon hunger is the downfall of the majority of my clients. The slow and steady decline, also known as the "diet witching hour," typically starts between three and five. By this time of day you're tired and stressed, and your blood sugar is crashing. As we saw in chapter 3, levels of neuropeptide Y start to rise, igniting your appetite for the complex carbs you need to replenish your depleted and tired body. A body that has run through its fuel supplies will release the stress hormone cortisol, which triggers the production and activity of this carb-craving hormone, as well as the fat-craving hormone galantin. As the cravings increase, especially for those bad boy foods, so do the unwanted pounds.

Fortunately, you can survive the diet witching hour with a few creative strategies:

Have a plan. Know what external cues set you off and be ready with a game plan. If, for example, holidays trigger overeating, consider bringing your own low-calorie food to the festivities. I have a client who always asks the host what she can bring to the party. This way, she gets to eat her own food but doesn't offend the host. I have another client who on her walk to work plans a route far away from the corner bakery and pizza parlor. Always make sure you have a low-calorie good guy alternative at your disposal when cravings strike. Try a piece of Sugar Blocker Gum or a Listerine Breath Strip, both of which are excellent for stopping cravings dead in their tracks.

Never eat when you're hungry. You know how doctors say that if you wait to drink until you're thirsty you're already dehydrated? The same goes for physical hunger. If you wait until you are physically hungry to eat, you're waiting too long. You need to eat before you get to that point. Otherwise, you'll eat with your eyes, and unlike our stomachs, they're bottomless pits.

Schedule your snack for the same time (or as close as possible) every afternoon. This way, your body will develop its own internal eating schedule, making it easier to recognize your own hunger cues.

Eat a high-fiber, high-protein snack. Fiber fills you up, and protein gives you staying power by helping to stabilize your blood sugar. Some of my Skinny Jeans Diet favorites include:

- Gnu Flavor and Fiber Bars, Clif KidZ Bars, Kashi Go Lean Protein and Fiber Bars
- An apple with one tablespoon of PB2 (powdered peanut butter)
- Dannon Light and Fit Greek Yogurt with one cup of berries
- A reduced-fat cheese stick, such as Sorrento or Weight Watchers, with an Emerald 100-calorie nut pack (be sure to buy the 100-calorie packs because nuts are naturally high in calories and you'll quickly lose count)
- Alba 70 Snack Shake Mix made with one cup of Almond Breeze Unsweetened Almond Milk
- Questbar
- Orville Reddenbacher's Smartpop! Popcorn 100-calorie mini-bags with a Laughing Cow Mini Babybel Cheese Round
- One Chocolite Protein Bar with an apple

Like Dorothy's ruby slippers, a healthy snack and a smart plan can revive your spirit and make you all-powerful against your food cravings. Over time, routine kicks in, and it gets easier and easier to douse those wicked witchy temptations.

What About PMS?

Portion-controlled snacking also works during that
time of the month right before your period when cravings are constant. Feeling premenstrual can lead even the most disciplined
dieter down the wrong path. Some of this is due to the placebo effect:
simply knowing you're getting your period makes you crave chocolate. But some of it is real too. When you have PMS, the feel-good
hormone serotonin is depressed. To compensate, you may crave
foods that help raise serotonin, such as sweets and simple carbs. Find
me a girl who hasn't run to chocolate at least once during that time
of the month. These foods quickly raise blood sugar, flood you with
insulin, and then send you crashing ignominiously to earth.

But you can use PMS to your advantage. A woman's basal metabolic rate rises 5 to 10 percent a few days before menstruation starts.
And while nothing in life is free, that does translate into getting a little
freebie in the calorie burn department. You burn anywhere from 75 to
150 extra calories a day the day or two prior to your period—*without
lifting a finger.* All good things must come to an end, however: once
you start menstruating, your metabolic rate returns to normal, or even
slightly less than normal.

Every woman has this cyclical metabolic rate, but the timing of the
rise and fall is different for each of us. If your periods are regular, you
can account for that dip in serotonin and increase in metabolic rate
with a well-timed, sensible plan. For example, if you know you always
crave chocolate the day before your period, go to the drugstore and
buy one chocolate bar that falls within the 75- to 150-calorie range. A
Nestlé 100 Baby Grand or a Ghirardelli Caramel Chocolate Bar both
clock in at 160 calories (close enough calorically in this case), and a
package of Pretzel M&Ms is 150 calories. The trick is to buy only one

single serving and to stop using your period as an excuse to eat, well, everything, for a week straight.

Distractions Work

ARE YOU A FOUR-ALARM-FIRE EATER? DOES EVEN THE SLIGHTEST hunger pang send you rushing to the nearest food source? Remember, a hunger pang isn't a green light to start shoveling food into your mouth. Rather, it's a gentle reminder to eat. In fact, studies show that most food urges, which are even stronger than cravings, subside within seven minutes.

My client Patricia recently shared an example of this distraction method. Patricia was part of a committee at work organizing a charity event to raise money for pediatric cancer. The head of the steering committee told Patricia that she was in charge of ordering a special blackout cake just for the event. After hearing this news, Patricia fantasized day and night about this cake. On the day of the event Patricia couldn't wait to taste a slice of that chocolate cake, but just as dessert was being served, a colleague cornered her about an upcoming deal. By the time they finished talking, the dessert had been cleared away. Though Patricia was momentarily annoyed at not having any cake, she realized that this work-related distraction had saved her several thousand calories and weeks' worth of uncontrollable cravings.

If you distract yourself from a food craving, it dissipates. Try to occupy your time; find a distracting activity such as cleaning out your junk drawer or reading *50 Shades of Grey* or a new magazine. Keep your mouth busy with a beverage, a piece of sugar-free gum, a lollipop, or a breath mint.

A NATURAL CRAVING-BUSTER SCENT

What's the most effective scent to help you sidestep cravings or fight off an all-out noshing bonanza? Peppermint! According to cutting edge research by Bryan Raudenbush, a leading researcher and assistant professor of psychology at Wheeling Jesuit University in West Virginia, subjects who sniffed mint periodically throughout the day ate 3,000 fewer calories over the course of a week (remember that 3,500 calories equals a pound)! Consider using peppermint gum, mini candy canes, scented candles, or hand lotion.

The Scan-and-Select Method

SPECIAL OCCASIONS CAN BE ESPECIALLY TRYING FOR THE CRAVING-challenged. Ever try staring down a half-dozen bad boyfriend–laden buffet tables? I advise clients who are worried about giving in to their baser instincts to try the scan-and-select strategy.

I have a client, Darcy, who loves those make-your-own-sundae bars. Nothing is off limits, including all those calorie-rich toppings. Darcy knew there would be a sundae bar at her friend's 40th birthday party. I asked Darcy: if she could use her calories on any one thing, what would it be? The answer came immediately: "I would give up all the other food if I could have a small double-mint-chip ice cream sundae."

"Do it," I told her. "Make that your selection and enjoy it to the fullest, provided it won't trigger overeating or cause you to start craving ice cream all the time."

This is a very common scenario in weight loss. Darcy didn't need to know the calories in her sundae. It was simple. We all know an iPad costs more than an iPhone, but we may not know the exact cost of all the different models or the different deals being offered at different retailers. Likewise, we all know an ice cream sundae has many more calories than grilled chicken skewers. If you check out all the food and then still indulge in a lavish dessert, chances are that you'll blow through an entire day's worth of calories in just one meal. Most important, Darcy knew herself. She knew that she could control the ice cream because she was eating it under controlled circumstances.

I have another client who was concerned about "blowing it" during her cousin's wedding. I advised her to carefully scan the food landscape and select the foods she could "buy" within her calorie "budget." I told her to walk around the cocktail-hour stations or wait a bit to see what hors d'oeuvres were being passed around. I always advise clients not to buy the first thing they see, since there might be something later on they like even more. Why pick up the first guy you meet at a bar when there's a chance George Clooney might walk through the door?

Once you decide on a few things you want to purchase with your calorie money, figure out which ones are the most valuable. Then "select" what you want to eat. If you don't see any food that turns you on as much as pigs in a blanket, then make that your choice (provided it's not a really bad boyfriend). Remember that pigs in a blanket are a high-calorie bite—and literally just a bite at that—so you won't have that much wiggle room for the rest of the night, which could leave you feeling deprived. You may want to ditch the pigs in favor of crudité and shrimp, which you can have a lot more of. You may also decide that the entrée choices aren't that appealing and choose a generous helping of salad instead, with the dressing on the side, which can save you a few hundred calories.

While a special event may not be a weight *loss* day, by scanning and selecting, you can enjoy your favorite foods without having to make it a weight *gain* day. This strategy is great for eliminating the feelings of deprivation that torment anyone trying to lose weight. If you opt for the scan-and-select strategy, be sure to reserve it for special occasions—it will backfire if used too often!

THE TWO-MINUTE PLAN

Did you know that on-the-spot temptations and food cravings derail 90 percent of dieters? Studies show that briefly tightening any group of muscles—your fist or shoulders, for example—can raise your craving resolve for up to two minutes, which is enough time to fight off any diet-sabotaging urge. Tensing your muscles subconsciously signals to your brain the need for more physical or mental strength in the moment. A big, gooey caramel chai latte would taste great, but you should ask yourself if you want it instead of your skinny jeans. A low-calorie skim milk cappuccino might not be quite as tasty, but nothing tastes worse than listening to yourself groan as you try to squeeze into your pants.

NINE WAYS TO KEEP THE CRAVING WOLVES AT BAY

Keep good company. Have an enjoyable good guy alternative as part of your daily food plan. In this case, an apple a day may help keep deprivation and cravings away!

Start a routine. Schedule your good guy food for the same time each day, such as a low-calorie frozen novelty after dinner. Here's the best part: on the Skinny Jeans Diet, you get a free 100 calories every night!

Keep it simple. Variety stimulates consumption. A little variety in your diet helps you avoid boredom, but too much variety stimulates cravings. For example, it may be good to have different protein choices for your meals, but to alternate between the same three snacks in the midafternoon. You don't want to get turned on by too many different tastes, textures, smells, and thoughts.

Distract for seven minutes. If you can distract yourself for seven minutes, most food cravings will pass! If you're concerned about heeding the clarion call of a bag of chips at the gas station food mart, then consider stopping at the dry cleaners before getting gas; then maybe a coffee will be all you grab when you fill your tank.

Don't bring bad boyfriends home. If you're concerned that a certain food will activate cravings, then don't let that naughty boy food back into your circle.

Out of sight isn't always out of mind. Throw problem foods into the trash bin or send them to work with your husband. But don't put them in the freezer. That won't save you from yourself. If they're within reach, you're in trouble. I have a client who would regularly munch on slightly defrosted cake.

Make them unappealing. Pour soap, salt, or pepper on the foods you're worried most about overeating.

Freshen your breath. Everybody hates to ruin a clean, cool mouth. Stick in a piece of sugar-free candy or gum, or make some cinnamon or peppermint tea to feel refreshed.

Drink something. Immediately after eating the food you were craving, cleanse your palate. Taste buds are satisfied in three bites, so washing the taste away helps the craving subside.

Grabbing the Bull by the Horns

It starts innocently enough. You're running errands at the local mall. You're there just to pick up a few items for your kids and a card for your mother's birthday. You swore that you'd be in and out in a couple of minutes max. Suddenly, a fancy display catches your eye. Those hot new designer shoes you've been eyeing for months are finally on sale. You turn away quickly, but they call to you. Within moments, you're in the store, credit card in hand, and next thing you know, you're walking out the door with your latest score, a lot lighter in the wallet and a lot heavier in guilt.

For many of us, a spur-of-the-moment shoe purchase isn't a big deal, but if you give in to every buying impulse, you'll quickly find yourself up to your eyeballs in debt. The fight you have with yourself to stop that urge can be worse than any fight you've ever had with your mother. It's no different in the world of food: the fight to resist cravings can be one of the toughest challenges you'll ever face. Keeping yourself from digging into your favorite food is no easy task, especially when you have the tag team of your neurochemistry and the 21st-century food environment vying for your attention.

This is why having a plan in place is critical to taking the reins of your cravings. Remember, cravings start in your head, not your belly. You can't always predict when a craving will hit, but you can always control your reaction. Have a plan in place for mastering tempting food situations, and learn exactly what you need to do to take back your craving control. Using the strategies in this chapter, you can keep a simple food craving from turning into a major diet disaster.

CHAPTER 6

Mistakes Are Meant to Teach Us

Oops! You did it again . . .

You know the scenario. You're losing weight and feeling good. You're approaching your diet goal and dreaming of that new red bikini you bought for your trip to Palm Beach. But then it happens: you slip. That single peanut butter cup you allow yourself as a treat quickly morphs into five or more. Perhaps you go out to dinner, tap into the bread basket, and can't stop. Or a bad day at the office causes your son's box of Devil Dogs to disappear. After a few days, you notice that you're a pound heavier. Your resolve weakens, causing you to slide even further. In no time flat, your weight is back where it started, and you feel like a big fat failure (literally).

This doesn't have to be your story. You can break through the "Oops, I did it again" cycle. A striking feature of the It Girls is that they don't procrastinate. In other words, they manage mistakes as soon as they occur. They monitor themselves closely, and if the scale starts to creep up, they immediately take the weight off. And on those rare occasions when the weight does come back, they have a set game plan for slimming down. Listen to the story of my It Girl client Jill, who has maintained her 20-pound weight loss for five years.

Jill's Story: Lasting Success

THOUGH TODAY SHE IS HAPPILY MARRIED, A SUCCESSFUL ENTRE-preneur, and the mother of three rambunctious teenage boys, Jill's life wasn't always a bed of roses. When Jill was 12, her mother died suddenly. "I started coming home to an empty house, and my playmates became a bag of pretzels or chips. My dad got takeout Chinese, pizza, or fast food for dinner most nights," she recalls. By the time she hit eighth grade, Jill clocked in at five-four and a hefty 160 pounds, which earned her the official designation of "fat girl."

Jill's dad tried to reassure her, telling her that she wasn't fat, just big-boned, and that she had a beautiful face. That wasn't going to cut it with Jill, who spent the next five years jumping from one diet to the next—all of which resulted in failure. After high school, she played around with popular diets, and she even created her own diets: eating nothing but fruit one day and protein the next. She would lose and regain the same 15 to 20 pounds. Her lifestyle was all or nothing—and completely unsustainable.

In college, Jill met her boyfriend (now husband). He ate healthily and loved to exercise. She started power-walking around her college campus. Her cooking became healthier, and she ate in smaller portions. As the weight went down, her self-esteem increased: her clothes fit, men did double takes, and most important, she felt happy and light. Her weight stabilized at 130 pounds—and it stayed there for a while.

By the time Jill turned 45, her age and new demands had taken their toll, and her weight had crept back up, to 150. She came to see me. After working out a structured meal plan, we got her back down to her college weight.

Today Jill starts her day with a sensible breakfast and brings lunch to work in her jewelry studio. She eats a plant-based diet, cooks healthily for her family, and keeps bad boyfriend foods out of her house. At three o'clock every afternoon, she indulges in a favorite treat: a "splash of skim" iced coffee with a high-fiber Gnu Bar. "It's become a ritual for me. I feel like I'm treating myself. It's my version of coffee and cake," says Jill. And it works.

To maintain her 20-pound weight loss, Jill steps on the scale every other day. If she hits 133, she's reached the top of her chosen weight range. This number is Jill's trigger to start snacking on fruit, weigh and measure her protein, and increase her nonstarchy vegetable intake. She will also eat the same thing for the next few days to recommit herself and deactivate cravings. She knows that her vigilance will cause her weight to go back down within three days.

Jill is confident that she can maintain her weight loss. She's learned through experience that if she gains a few pounds, she can lose them again by cutting back right away—rather than going to an extreme. Timeliness is of utmost importance.

In a recent session, I asked her if it was difficult to maintain this lifestyle change now that the newness had faded. She thought about it carefully. "My biggest hurdle was learning to add structure to my eating. I'll always remember where I came from, and be happy and proud of where I am. I focus on how good that feels, and how much I enjoy getting dressed. These reminders feel fresh every day—and they are priceless," she said.

It Girls Make Mistakes, Too

It Girls make mistakes too. But when they do, they are the opposite of victims: they are women of action and resolve. If and when they hit the top of their weight range, they get busy. They don't let the weight gain give them any excuses, and they don't come up with "convenient" reasons for their failure.

Like Jill, It Girls manage their mistakes meal by meal and day by day. If they overate at lunch, they have a dinner of steamed vegetables. If they went overboard at a wedding buffet, they cut back the next day or two. They keep their weight within a weight range, usually within one to five pounds. They know that reversing small weight gains immediately is one of the most important skills they can learn and need to practice . . . permanently.

This is not to say that you need to take drastic measures. You may just need to return to basics, going back to your regular way of eating and letting the extra pounds take care of themselves. As my client Jen says, "I go back to the Skinny Jeans Diet basics if I see a pound or two creep up."

The It Girls are action-oriented. If they hit the top of their weight range, they do something about it. They are obstinate about establishing and keeping a maximum upper limit for weight. They don't hold a pity party, brood over it, or sit around passively, but rather get on it. Within a short time, their weight is back down to the lower end of their weight range.

When you make a weight loss mistake, instead of viewing your actions as pain and punishment, put a more positive spin on them. Remind yourself that it takes a lot less energy to deal with five pounds than with 10, 20, or 30 pounds. Focus on how good—even ecstatic—

you feel when you're in control of your food. Think about how much fun it will be to hit a farmers' market, try a new low-calorie recipe, and get those hot leather pants to button.

IS "BAD" THE NEW "GOOD?"

Are you having two slices of birthday cake, finishing your child's French fries, and topping your frozen yogurt with crushed Oreos? Most dieters think that being "bad" will feel "good," but science says the opposite may be true. It turns out that cavorting with your bad boyfriend foods after a week of keeping company with salads and hitting the gym is even worse for your psyche than expected.

In a groundbreaking food and mood study published in the prestigious *American Journal of Clinical Nutrition*, 160 women tracked what they ate for 10 days. Every two hours, a researcher contacted each woman to learn what she'd just eaten and how she felt about it. The researchers considered two variables: (1) how the meal compared to the subject's typical meal (more healthy or more indulgent?), and (2) whether the meal was eaten at home or at a restaurant, café, or friend's house.

By and large, the women were significantly happier and calmer after eating healthier, lower-calorie meals, and eating them at home, where they had control over the choices, ingredients, and method of preparation.

Instead of reveling in the short-term rewards, they

took solace in meeting long-term goals. Rather than getting charged up by their indulgences, they took pride in their successes. So take a second look at your favorite bad boyfriend indulgence and ask yourself if it really makes you happy. You might be surprised by the answer.

One Mistake Does Not a Diet Break

LOSING WEIGHT IS A LIFESTYLE CHANGE, AND ONE THAT CAN BE hard to make, let alone maintain. When you lapse, you do something unplanned and unintended that makes you feel guilty. That's not great for weight control, but it's also *not* a reason to throw in the towel.

A lapse can take a number of different forms. Maybe you grabbed a Hershey's Kiss out of your colleague's candy jar on impulse, or took a bagel off the breakfast tray at the school PTA meeting. Maybe you downed an entire sub at your daughter's birthday party—or binged in solitude one idle night. Whatever it was, it was *not* on your to-do list for that day. (If you plan an indulgence, it's not a mistake—it's a treat that has been accounted for and balanced within the context of your larger eating schedule.)

Viewing the occasional mistake as a learning experience can keep it from growing into something even larger. Think about what went wrong and how you can prevent a similar situation in the future. Then—most important—forgive yourself. Tell yourself that everyone makes mistakes and it's time to carry on.

The problem is that dieters go overboard. They become perfectionists and treat their mistakes as personal indications of failure. It's an unforgiving, defeatist attitude, and it can only lead to bigger problems.

Let's say that, after a month of following a low-calorie diet, you give in at a favorite restaurant. The next day you skip breakfast to make up for your transgression—and by noon you're famished. *Screw it*, you think, and you order pizza, grilled cheese, or onion rings. Now it's more than a single, isolated mistake. You've embarked on a series of mistakes and are on the brink of trashing your diet and gaining all of that poundage back. That, my girlfriends, is the *real* mistake.

Mistakes aren't personal. They don't label you as weak. They're just a particular response to an independent situation. And yes, they *can* be reversed.

The Journey to Thin

SOMETIMES LOSING WEIGHT FEELS SO HARD. YOU THINK, *THIS IS too much work, I don't have it in me.* You're momentarily disappointed or feeling deprived, frustrated, and impatient.

At that precise moment, the cravings for your old food ways begin, undermining your desire to continue to care for yourself in your new way. You start to think that your old destructive behaviors and food choices will help you feel better. You venture into risky territory by doing something like agreeing to meet a friend for coffee . . . at your favorite bakery. In *Growing Ourselves Up: A Guide to Recovery and Self-Esteem,* author Stanley J. Gross, Ed.D., says, "At some point after making a change, the demands of maintaining it seem to outweigh the benefits of the change. We don't remember that this is normal. Change involves resistance."

Preventing one mistake from derailing you entirely requires a smart action plan. Have an action plan ready to go—and use it when it's needed. For instance, have a plan to:

- Call a friend
- Slowly back away from the food
- Write in your food diary about what you're feeling
- Remind yourself how far you've come—and acknowledge it
- Reach out to your nutritionist or other support person or group
- Review the basics of your diet plan
- Eat a low-calorie food until the urge for the tempting one passes (think carrots with salsa versus leftover pasta)

If we understand that making a mistake is a natural result of our resistance to change, we'll be able to go back to our diet with minimal guilt and lots of confidence to keep moving forward. Here's how to get your thinking back on track:

1. **Congratulate yourself on your awareness of the mistake.** Plenty of dieters make them—and neglect to pause and assess. Take time to pat yourself on the back, because this is the beginning of a long, productive ride. Every time you catch a mistake and nip it in the bud, you increase your skill set. You get another notch on your mistake experience belt, and you build your confidence going forward.

2. **Think about how you became vulnerable, and zap the threat of it happening again.** See what set you up and compare it to mistakes you may have made in the past. Does grocery shopping prompt you to eat bad boy foods—directly out of the cart? One solution might be to do your food shopping online, *after* you've eaten, or send your spouse to the market the next time. Was it the smell of fries at McDonald's? Next time take the kids through the drive-thru to prevent risky situations—ahead of time.

   My client Stacy, a nurse at a busy metropolitan-area hospital, is known for going the extra mile with her patients. They often thank her with homemade baked goods. Around the holidays, it's not uncommon for her to get tins filled with cakes, chocolate-covered marshmallows, cookies, and muffins. One day she had a slipup involving a box of rainbow cookies. I asked her to formulate a strategy for the next time. She said she'd eat just one, then immediately gift the cookies to a nursing station on another floor, or to the housekeeping staff. Since this one slipup, it hasn't been an issue for Stacy.

   Your goal isn't to fix every situation or be perfect every second of every day. Your goal is to manage and limit your risk. Try to anticipate the situation, apply the coping skills you find most helpful, and keep in mind that mistakes will happen.

3. **Cope with the threat head-on.** You can't eliminate all high-risk situations, but you *can* learn to handle them more effectively when they happen. If parties are your downfall,

realize that it's unrealistic to stay away from them. See page 150 for some suggestions on how to navigate parties—and stick to your guns.

My client Karen struggles with weekends. She wants to eat everything: her kids' pizza, the bread in the Saturday night bread basket, and both the bagels *and* the cream cheese at the bagel store. To her the weekend isn't fun without eating her way through it. We couldn't eliminate the weekends, but we *could* devise a structured weekend food plan that incorporated Karen's social plans. I suggested to Karen that she stay out of the kitchen weekend afternoons and busy herself during that time. Maybe take in a movie (and be sure to bring her own popcorn), run errands, go for a walk. Anything to distract her from mindless eating. I also suggested that she drink lots of cold water, which has been shown to reduce appetite. We kept her busy and structured—and it worked.

Your strategy might be behavioral (walk away from the food, distract yourself with another activity, call a friend, eat a low-calorie food until the urge passes) or cognitive (give yourself a pep talk, acknowledge your successes, meditate). Whenever I walk into my house at the end of the day, my thoughts automatically go to food. While I can't avoid coming home, I have trained myself to walk right past the kitchen and up to my bedroom to change into my loungewear (behavioral strategy), which gives me time to unwind without using food as a crutch. I also use that time to think about the consequences of overeating (cognitive strategy). By the time I enter the kitchen, I am ready for something healthy, like an apple or peach from the huge fruit bowls I keep on the counter (behavioral strategy) versus chips, dips, or nuts.

4. **Forgive and move on.** This is the most important one. Okay, you overate . . . *a lot.* Don't berate yourself. Just begin again. If you wallow in guilt, it will cause you to eat even more.

Get Real

HAVE YOU EVER SWORN OFF CHOCOLATE FOR THE REST OF YOUR life? Or declared your intention to lose two pounds a week? Maybe you've opted to boycott all birthday celebrations at the office—indefinitely.

If this sounds familiar, it's time to take a page from Dr. Phil and "get real." Making unrealistic goals and pledges sets you up to fail.

Unlike many dieters, It Girls set manageable, attainable goals. Instead of going from A to Z, they go from A to G, and then from G to M, and then from M to Z. They accomplish their objectives over the course of time, and they celebrate their progress along the way. If your downfall is doughnuts, consider enjoying one every Sunday with your kids in the park versus swearing them off completely. Getting real requires you to change things moderately and gently—not radically. If you always gain weight on vacation, then don't vow to lose weight the next time you're away; just strive to maintain. If you wind down every night with a snack in front of the TV, don't stop. Just make sure the snack is a good guy food, and good for your diet.

WORKING IN PAIRS

Similar to being realistic is being specific.

Vague goals tend to fail because they're impossible to measure. Rather than creating vague goals, set two specific goals for each day and two specific goals for each week. Ask yourself what's reasonable. Rather than vowing to eat "less" after dinner (vague), opt to clean and leave the kitchen by eight o'clock (specific), with a 100-calorie ice cream sandwich in hand (specific).

Other examples include:

DAILY GOALS

1. Eat fruit as a mid-morning snack to replace that starchy snack.

2. Get out of the kitchen by eight o'clock at night—and don't look back.

WEEKLY GOALS

1. Go to the farmers' market by your office and stock up on produce for the week.

2. Cook roasted vegetables in batches on the weekends to eat all week long.

MONTHLY GOALS

1. Focus on losing five pounds (more manageable) rather than 20 pounds (overwhelming).

2. Get to bed earlier, since people who get more sleep lose more weight.

See the Forest for the Trees

To lose weight and keep it off, you have to make lifestyle changes. This may mean adjusting your meal schedule, checking menus online, addressing your feelings more effectively, and shopping and cooking differently. When your success at weight loss is the result of meeting many small, achievable goals, it becomes more difficult for you to point to any single slipup as a mistake. *One mistake doesn't undo all of your positive changes.*

I asked Jill (whose success story I shared on page 119) what her secret is. "I don't beat myself up. I don't obsess. I put everything in perspective. After years of struggle, I finally see the big picture. One brownie won't erase my healthy lifestyle, and a pack of gummy bears won't eliminate my daily practices," she said. "Nor would I allow that."

I couldn't have said it better.

CHAPTER 7

Food Situations: Mastering Your Food Universe

B Y NOW YOU'VE IDENTIFIED YOUR BAD BOYFRIEND FOODS. You've learned the secrets of the It Girls. You've discovered that your troubled relationship with food isn't entirely your fault. You've taken the emotion out of emotional eating. And you know how to beat back the most devastating chocolate cravings.

Eating is one of life's most enjoyable activities. Thus, this chapter is all about having fun while keeping yourself firmly in check. First, I'll talk about everyday food situations: dining out, weekends, food shopping, entertaining, and living in a house full of food. Next, I'll walk you through those less frequent events such as holidays, parties, traveling, and vacations.

As I've repeated throughout this book, we inhabit a world that seems to want nothing more than to make us fat. We cannot escape our 24/7 world of food—we have to coexist with food—but with the right strategies, we can handle any and every situation in our lives with confidence, dignity, and grace.

Dining Out

IT USED TO BE THAT EATING AT HOME WAS THE NORM AND DINING out was a special treat. Not anymore. If you eat in a restaurant four times a week, congratulations—you're officially an average American. Unfortunately, the average American is also overweight or obese.

Luckily, dining out doesn't have to doom your diet. I have clients who eat at fine restaurants every night but still manage to lose weight and maintain their weight loss. These days you can have your cake and eat it too by following a few creative strategies.

DOES EATING OUT MAKE YOU HAPPIER?

Researchers who looked at restaurant meals versus healthy, home-cooked meals found that women are significantly happier and less stressed after eating at home and after eating healthier meals. It seems that the home is often a sacred environment that feels cozy and nurtures healthy eating and healthier food choices. This makes us feel better about our food choices, which makes us feel better overall.

Does that mean you should say no to going out to eat? Of course it doesn't. It just means you have to be smart when eating out so that you'll leave the restaurant feeling happier instead of heavier. What could be better than that?

Simple Rules for Eating Out

To stay in control when eating out, follow these tips:

1. **It starts with the waiter!** This is my very best restaurant tip. Place your order how you intend to eat it. If the menu says the sea bass entrée comes with both polenta and sautéed spinach, omit the heavy carbs. Order it with a double portion of steamed or lightly sautéed spinach. That moment when you place your order sets you up for success (or lack of it) for the whole meal.

2. **Never give yourself the benefit of the doubt.** Don't try to convince yourself that you're only going to eat two or three of the fries that come with the burger you ordered sans bun. You know from past experience that this doesn't happen. Substitute a side of broccoli, tomato slices, or the vegetable of the day for the fries. It's easier to make a good choice when the bad one isn't sitting right in front of you.

3. **Do your homework.** Always check the restaurant menu online before going out so you'll have an idea of what you'll eat before arriving hungry at the restaurant. You want to make a smart choice based on your brain, not your belly.

4. **Vegetables should take up the most real estate on your plate.** Order a double portion of vegetables with your meal, preferably steamed. Or, if you want to mix a little sautéed vegetable with your steamed, order some sautéed

vegetables to share with your dinner companions. Then cover your plate of steamed vegetables with some of the table's sautéed vegetables to give yourself a little bit of flavor without all the hidden calories.

5. **Order two appetizers.** The portion sizes at some restaurants are staggering, and it's easy to overeat by a few hundred calories based on portion size alone. That's why I counsel clients to order two appetizers instead of a main course. It's one of the best forms of portion control I know of. But have the waiter bring the appetizers separately; otherwise, you may feel as if you're missing out. Imagine staring into space for an hour while your dining companions leisurely finish their meal.

6. **Be creative.** Mix and match different ingredients on the menu to make a healthy meal. Do you want the sea bass that comes with rice pilaf served with the Brussels sprouts that come with the pasta primavera instead? Just ask. Then leave a nice tip.

7. **End the meal with a hot, low-calorie beverage.** It will keep your hands and mouth busy. Coffee, tea, or hot water with lemon is available at every restaurant.

8. **Don't start.** If there's a bad boyfriend food on the table, ask the waiter to remove it or move it out of view and arm's reach. For many ladies, that first bite is all it takes to trigger an avalanche. One study found that diners at

Italian restaurants eat hundreds of calories in bread and oil before the meal is even served.

9. **Keep your salad skinny.** Add-ins like bacon, cheese, croutons, nuts, and dried fruit can ruin the best salad intentions.

10. **Ask for dressings and sauces on the side, please!** Always ask for high-calorie sauces and dressings to be served on the side. Use a fork, not a spoon, to dribble the dressing on top, or just dip.

11. **Don't be afraid to ask.** Do tell the waiter exactly how you want your food prepared. Ask about the ingredients and how the food is usually prepared. If the restaurant allows it, you can even make up your own meal combinations from different menu items.

12. **Nix the prix fixe.** "Prix fixe" is another way of saying "supersize me." Here's the other thing to consider—if you're paying for the food, you may feel compelled to eat it all.

13. **Avoid surprises.** Don't let a night of dining out turn a meal that's grilled or roasted into a meal that's grilled with oil or roasted with butter. Chefs often add a pat of butter under the skin of chicken or on top of a steak to give it a glaze. Ask for your food "grilled with very little oil" and request your steak sans butter.

Around the World in Skinny Jeans

I TOOK A FEW POPULAR RESTAURANT TYPES—CHINESE, JAPANESE, Italian, Indian, Mexican, and fast-food—and figured out how to navigate them. Follow these rules and you can't go wrong!

STIR-FRY SURVIVAL KIT

Chinese food is a very interesting cuisine. While many of the dishes are rich in lean protein and have a high volume of vegetables, those same dishes also contain too much oil and cornstarch-thickened sauce. Here's the best way to choose Chinese.

1. **Start with soup.** Choosing a broth-based soup can fill you up while reducing your total meal calories. Chinese soup stats:
    - Egg drop soup: 65 calories and 3 grams of fat per 1 cup
    - Hot and sour soup: 75 calories and 3 grams of fat per 1 cup
    - Wonton soup: 140 calories and 5 grams of fat per 1 cup (1 wonton)

2. **Steam it.** It's the only way to go when eating Chinese food on the Skinny Jeans Diet. You can get steamed veggie dumplings, steamed shrimp and broccoli, or any other lean protein or veggie dish steamed and served with sauce on the side. Just dip your fork into the sauce and dribble it over your food.

3. **Opt for the lowest-calorie sauce.** Black bean is best, and ask for it on the side.

4. **Watch the rice.** If you do decide to eat rice, fill your teacup with it: that's a half-cup serving. Give the remainder to your dining companions or send it immediately back to the kitchen with your waiter.

5. **Use your chopsticks.** Not too skilled at it? All the better! The point of using these tricky sticks is to slow you down. Eating more slowly allows your stomach to process the food you've already eaten, so your brain gets the message that you're fuller faster.

6. **Enjoy your fortune.** A fortune cookie is a great way to end your meal with a little sweetness and not a lot of calories. Fortune cookies are fat-free, with 30 calories each.

7. **Avoid *all* of the following:**
    - *Egg rolls:* One large egg roll has about 350 calories and 15 grams of fat—and it's just an appetizer!
    - *Egg foo young:* One meal has about 600 calories and 40 grams of fat.
    - *Fried rice:* One cup of this fatty side dish contains 400 calories and 13 grams of fat.
    - *General Tso's chicken:* One cup of this favorite fried dish has about 390 calories and 17 grams of fat.
    - *Kung pao chicken:* We're talking 500 calories and 26 grams of fat. Avoid, avoid, avoid!!

Turning Japanese—And Staying on Track

Japanese food can be a great way to stay slim while dining out. But there are pitfalls. Below is a short list to help steer you in the right direction.

1. **As with Chinese food, start with soup.** Miso soup has about 50 calories per cup, so use that to take the edge off your appetite.

2. **Beware of edamame.** It's a healthy starter, and packed with protein and fiber. However, a half-cup shelled serving contains 130 calories. Be careful if you still have a meal coming.

3. **Love your sashimi.** This is a great-tasting, protein-rich fish or seafood meal sans rice. On the Skinny Jeans Diet, you can have eight pieces for dinner or lunch.

4. **Ask for your sushi with "light" rice.** No, that isn't brown rice. It's just having less rice, literally.

5. **Beware of the calories in a sushi roll.** That rice is packed tight. One California roll typically has 280 to 300 calories.

6. **Order rolls "Naruto style."** That means the roll is wrapped in cucumber instead of rice. This is a great alternative that is high-volume and low-calorie. You can order one roll regular style and one roll Naruto style.

You'll get lots of pieces of sushi, but drastically cut down on the calories.

Great choices:

- *Cucumber roll:* This roll has 130 calories and no fat.
- *Spicy tuna roll:* If it doesn't have too much mayo, one roll has 250 to 290 calories and 5 to 10 grams of fat.
- *California roll:* Order one without mayo for a 275- to 300-calorie count and 5- to 10-gram fat count.
- Steamed *lettuce wraps:* The traditional dish is close to 900 calories. Order this wrap steamed with the hoisin sauce on the side. Just dribble the sauce over the diced filling and your dish will come in just under 300 calories. Plus, lettuce wraps require assembly, which slows down the meal.

7. **Add vegetables to your sushi meal.** Try *oshitashi* (boiled spinach with soy sauce) or cucumber *sunomono* (sweet cucumber salad made with rice vinegar).
   - *Tempura:* Japanese for "batter-fried"
   - *Spider rolls:* Greasy, fried crab rolls
   - *Dynamite:* Sushi-speak for "mayo"
   - *Crunch:* Sushi-speak for "fried"

MAMMA MIA! DIETING IN ITALIAN

Think Italian food, and pasta and pizza usually spring to mind first. But luckily, the Mediterranean cuisine also encompasses rich soups, antipasto, meat, and fish. Italian cooks love their (healthy but high-calorie) olive oil, so be careful when ordering.

1. **Avoid the bread basket.** The aroma alone can make you want to eat every last piece. Italian bread contains hundreds of calories and loads of fat (it's usually made with oil). Ask for it not to be brought to the table in the first place.

2. **Start with steamed mussels or clams.** This appetizer will keep your hands busy while your companions dine on easier-to-eat fried calamari and mozzarella sticks.

3. **Steer clear of pasta-based dishes.** If there's a pasta dish you must have, ask that it be made in an appetizer-size portion. Lean toward red, clam, or meatless marinara sauces—and away from Alfredo, meat, and carbonara sauces.

4. **Order thin crust or** margherita **pizza.** You'll save hundreds of calories on the crust alone. When you get your pizza, remove half the cheese and use your fork to spread what's left over the entire slice.

5. **Try dishes like chicken, seafood, or veal cacciatore or** pizzaiola. Even better are grilled white fishes such as *branzino*. Ask that it be broiled or grilled *without* butter or oil.

6. **Request a steamed vegetable for yourself and a sautéed vegetable for the table.** Take some of the sautéed veggie and spread it over your steamed veggie. You get some of the flavor without all the calories.

EATING INDIAN: HAVE YOUR NAAN—AND EAT IT TOO

The land that invented yoga is also a booby trap filled with naan, heavy curries, roti, and Samosa. What's a Skinny Jeans Dieter to do? I'll tell you!

1. **As with Chinese and Japanese, start with soup.** A cup of lentil soup (about 130 calories and 3 grams of fat) is packed with protein and fiber and can fill you up so that you eat less at your meal.

2. **Quarter your naan—or skip it entirely.** Naan bread is cooked in a tandoori oven. It's a pillowy-soft accompaniment for your curry or other entrée, but just one piece of this buttery side dish contains 580 calories and 20 grams of fat. Stick to one quarter and you're still looking at 145 calories of bread. If bread is a bad boyfriend food for you, don't even start. Safer bet: order some saffron rice for the table and spread two teaspoons over your dish for fewer calories (about 75)—and zero bread compulsion.

3. **For your main course, tandoori chicken or fish is the way to go.** It's basically roasted meat marinated in yogurt and spices.
   - *Chicken or fish tikka:* This dish is very similar to tandoori, although avoid cream-based tikka masala.
   - *Skip lamb and beef* to watch calories and fat.
   - *Beware of anything with a curry sauce.* It's made from coconut milk, flour, and butter.

4. **Don't assume that vegetables are your friends.** A lot of people think vegetables are okay, no matter what the environment. In Indian food, many vegetables are laden with cheese, potatoes, and heavy sauces. Not sure about a vegetable dish? Ask your server how it's prepared.

5. **Pass on puri.** It's deep-fried flatbread.

6. **Spice things up.** Indian food can be spicy, which is nice in two ways. First, some experts say that spicy foods give our metabolism a temporary boost (helping to burn off some of the meal we are eating). Second, there is evidence that spiciness causes us to eat less, as we don't need to eat as much to experience the full flavor.

DON'T LET YOUR WAISTLINE GO SOUTH OF THE BORDER: EATING MEXICAN

Ay, caramba! Mexican food can be loaded with calories. So be careful and don't let Taco Tuesdays turn into Can't Zip Your Jeans Wednesdays!

1. **Where to start? Not with that basket of chips and guacamole!** You can easily eat 500 calories before your meal even hits the table. Start with seviche—fresh seafood in citrus juice with chopped veggies. Or order salad and use the salsa as your salad dressing.

2. **Double up!** Order two soft tacos, but eat only one tortilla. Combine the fillings of the two tacos, get rid of the extra tortilla, and have one big, huge taco.

3. **Avoid slippery slides.** Avoid oil- and butter-laden sides like rice, refried beans, cheese, guacamole, and tortilla chips. Instead, ask for veggies, plain black beans, salad (dressing on the side), salsa, *pico de gallo,* and taco sauce.

4. **Love fajitas.** Order a shrimp, chicken, or beef fajita cooked with very little oil. Skip the sides such as sour cream, guacamole, and refried beans. Instead, ask for extra peppers and onions. Stuff one or two of the corn tortillas to the brim and eat the rest open-faced.

5. **Watch the shell.** Order the popular taco salad in a ceramic bowl instead of the shell "bowl," which can set you back 400 calories!

6. **Be your own bartender.** Did you know there are usually 350 to 450 calories in a margarita? Order a tequila with water or club soda and sneak in a packet of Crystal Light Sugar-Free Lemonade or Margarita-Flavored Drink Mix. Save hundreds of calories.

Fast Food: Avoiding a Diet Minefield

Who doesn't want a toy with their hamburger? Who would turn down lunch in a 1950s-style diner? Who on earth can resist the smell of McDonald's French fries?

Fast food is inexpensive, convenient, and fun. And to many, it tastes very good. It's also low in nutrition and high in sodium and fat, and just one fast-food meal can pack enough calories for an entire day.

But fast food doesn't have to wreak havoc on your diet. Choose wisely and you can find some fast-food gems. Most of the major chains have responded to the call for healthy food by adding salads or salad bars, soups, reduced-fat sandwiches, and fruit options. Some also provide nutritional fact brochures on their websites and menus, so it's easy to be strategic. If you do some advance planning, a fast-food restaurant should be no different than any other eating-out situation. Here are some tips for navigating a fast-food nation:

1. **Bring your own portable meal, then use the drive-thru window only for kids' meals.** This can help you avoid the temptations you might encounter if you went inside the restaurant.

2. **If you need to step inside, follow my lead.** On nights I know we will be eating fast food, I am often seen bringing (okay, sneaking) my own food bag into the fast-food restaurant so that I have something healthy and low-fat of my own to eat.

3. **Don't fall into the trap of finishing your kids' leftovers.**
   Order a salad or healthy side dish so your mouth is busy
   while the kids are eating.

4. **"Undress" your food.** When choosing items, be aware of
   calorie- and fat-packed salad dressings, spreads, cheese,
   sour cream, and so on. For example, ask for a grilled
   chicken salad without the pecans or cranberries or bacon
   bits. You can also ask for the diet salad dressing packet.

5. **Special-order.** Many menu items could be healthy if it
   weren't for the way they were prepared. Ask for a grilled
   chicken sandwich without the mayonnaise. You can ask
   for a packet of ketchup or mustard and add it yourself,
   controlling how much you put on your sandwich.

6. **Find your inner child.** Ordering from the kids' menu can
   give you forced portion control. A Burger King Whopper
   with a small order of fries is an 800-calorie meal, yet a kids'
   meal hamburger and fries is a 300-calorie meal. To make
   the meal even lighter, take off the top bun and eat the
   burger open-faced and order apple slices instead of fries.

7. **Do not supersize—ever—no matter how good a "deal"
   it seems to be.** A typical single supersize serving provides
   1,000 calories—enough for *two* meals.

8. **Practice fowl play.** Chicken dishes often seem like the most diet-friendly choice, but at many chains you'll find lower-calorie options elsewhere on the menu. At McDonald's, the Premium Grilled Chicken Classic Sandwich is 350 calories, while the hamburger is 250 calories. At Au Bon Pain, the Chicken Cobb Salad is 660 calories, while the Tuna Garden Salad is 400 calories.

9. **Say no to the all-you-can-eat-buffet.** Even potentially healthy buffets, such as salad bars, can tempt us with too much variety. You're also likely to overeat when trying to get your money's worth. If you do choose the buffet, resist the temptation to go for seconds. Even better, order off the menu.

10. **Get on the health bandwagon.** Most chains have healthy menu options that feature less fat and fresher ingredients. Look for them.

11. **Beware of feeling virtuous.** While many sub shops, such as Subway, promote the health benefits of eating their food, studies have found that people eat more calories per meal at a sub shop than at McDonald's. This may be because you feel so virtuous eating "healthy," as their ads suggest, that you reward yourself with chips, extra condiments, or higher-calorie menu selections that can turn a good meal bad fast. Use common sense to make healthier choices. Just asking the server to "scoop" out the inside of the hero bread can cut about 200 calories!

12. **Pick any of my Skinny Jeans Diet fast-food special winners:**

   - *Healthiest fast-food hamburger:* McDonald's (260 calories, 9 grams fat) or Wendy's Jr. (280 calories, 9 grams fat)
   - *Healthiest fast food, Mexican:* Taco Bell taco salad without the shell, sour cream, or cheese (330 calories, 13 grams fat)
   - *Healthiest fried chicken:* KFC Original Recipe breast with breading and skin removed, and a side of green beans (190 calories, 4.5 grams fat) or KFC grilled chicken thigh and a small side of corn on the cob (240 calories, 10 grams fat)
   - *Healthiest sub chain sub:* Subway six-inch roast beef sub on whole wheat bread with veggies and honey mustard, no mayo (290 calories, 5 grams fat)
   - *Healthiest fast-food pizza:* Two slices of Pizza Hut Fit 'N Delicious Chicken and Veggie Pizza (208 calories, 9 grams fat)

The Weekends: Plan W

WEEKENDS CAN BE CHALLENGING FOR DIETERS. YOU'VE GOT LAZY days, late-night dinners, and unstructured time. But you've also got a calendar full of activities and social events. Often we gain back what we lose during the week on the weekends and find ourselves forever playing catchup with the scale. What's the solution to this nasty cycle?

Forget plan A or plan B and develop a Plan W for the weekend! A flexible but structured weekend plan is imperative. It's the best way I know to fight off the Monday blues.

1. **Make the weekends count.** Plan activities and cook healthy foods for the week ahead. Just don't put off your weight loss program for two whole days, or you'll wind up putting on the weight!

2. **Be smart on Sunday.** Make Sunday the day to get organized for the next few days. Get your food supplies, plot your weekly meals, and decide on a goal for the week. Planning ahead on Sunday makes Monday, Tuesday, and Wednesday a lot more diet-friendly.

3. **Have a splurge meal (or day).** Plan one meal a week that is a splurge meal, and use it on the weekend if that makes the most sense for your social schedule.

4. **Don't give back all you worked so hard for during the week.** Structure your weekend and plan for special social events. If weekend afternoon downtime is your challenge, see a matinee movie or schedule your errands for that time so you're not hanging around the house being tempted to snack. Look over all your weekend plans on Friday and figure out where you'll indulge and where you'll pull back.

Food Shopping Strategies: Having a "Smart Cart"

YOU CAN'T EAT YOUR BAD BOYFRIEND FOODS AT HOME ON THE weekends if you don't buy your bad boyfriend foods at the supermarket. And since the majority of our overeating is done in the comfort of our own kitchen, shopping smart is of vital importance. No excuses. Here are some strategies to making your cart smart.

1. **Don't shop hungry.** You'll shop with your belly instead of your brain. You need to have your wits about you to resist your bad boyfriends!

2. **Stick to your list.** Sticking to your list will help you put the supplies you need for success in the cart and leave out the ones you definitely don't need. If you don't have a list, now is a good time to make one. Don't wait!

3. **Skinny starts in the cart.** Every It Girl I know has a "smart cart" and fills it with foods she doesn't have a history of overeating. No bad boyfriend foods are allowed in a smart cart. If it follows you home, you will eat it. Period.

4. **Say no to sample sales.** Who doesn't love four designer sweaters for the price of one? In the world of food, sample sales will leave you bankrupt. When you walk by those small stands giving out free samples, just remember—a cheese cube here and a chip with salsa there really do add up. Even a small cheese cube can add 100 calories to your

diet—and do you really want to spend those calories on some random cheese in the grocery store? Many of my clients find that chewing gum while they shop helps them avoid sample snacking. Alternatively, shop during non-mealtime hours, as samples are not given out as plentifully then. If you still need a deterrent, remember that many sample foods have been sitting exposed on open plates for hours and it takes just 10 minutes for potentially dangerous bacteria to settle on food. This may be one sample sale worth passing on.

5. **Shop online.** If supermarket shopping is crushing your skinny jeans dreams, try shopping online to reduce temptation. Fresh Direct, Whole Foods, and Peapod are great grocery delivery options.

Smart Socializing

WHETHER YOU'RE HOSTING A BIG BASH FOR 200 OR A DINNER PARTY for 20, parties should be a blast. Everyone should be able to attend a festivity—or host one herself—without worrying about weight gain and too-tight pants. With the right strategies, parties can be fun, not fattening.

If You're the Host . . .

1. **Treat the occasion as an isolated event when buying food for company.** You may have foods in the house that aren't usually there, and this may lead to overeating. Buy as close to the exact amount of the food items you need and, if possible, try to make those purchases only one or two days in advance. So, if you're hosting a small family party and cake is your issue, consider buying a single cupcake for each guest (and sending any leftover cupcakes home with your guests).

2. **If your menu calls for a bad boyfriend food, keep it out of sight until it's time to cook or serve.** I have a client who squirreled away her husband's birthday cake in a neighbor's refrigerator. If you're having the food catered and there will be some bad boyfriends in the mix, make sure the caterer delivers your goodies at the last possible moment.

3. **Keep it simple and plan ahead.** Your menus should be simple, and you should plan in advance what you're going to cook and serve. Lack of planning leads to panic, worrying, and impulse buying, all of which can lead you back into the arms of the bad boyfriend you've been trying to avoid. Calm and collected dieters keep emotional eating to a minimum.

4. **Be vigilant.** As a host, you tend to relax once you see that your event is a success and your guests are having fun. Relief and happiness can cause you to overeat just as much as tension. Don't start picking.

5. **Be wary of mindless eating.** I can't tell you how many clients, especially if they're hosting the big shindig, unconsciously pop little bits of food into their mouths. Before too long, those little bits can add up to an entire meal (and then some). If this is your habit, prepare a plate for yourself, cover it with plastic wrap, and sit down and enjoy your meal when there's a lull in the evening or at the end of the party. Of course, few of us can wait that long to eat, especially when there's food all around. An even better option is to put aside a plate of low-calorie finger foods that you can dip into when hunger surfaces, such as cut-up vegetables, low-fat cheese cubes, bruschetta (dry toast is hard to abuse), a high-fiber cracker such as GG Bran Crispbread, or shrimp cocktail.

6. **Don't let them leave your home without it.** If you're serving a special food in honor of a guest, it should go home with that person, especially if it's something that might tempt you. I have a client who hands out doggie bags to her guests. If there's still some food left over, throw it out immediately. You're tough, but you may be no match for a half-empty plate of chocolate chip cookies. Don't put yourself in a compromising position.

7. **Ask for help.** If there's a bad boyfriend food you *must* serve at an event, ask someone else to prepare and bring it. It will be easier to separate from a food, even a bad boyfriend, that you didn't invest any time, effort, or money in. I always farm out dessert, especially baked goods, since that is my Achilles' heel. I don't want to see it days before a party or have it loitering around my kitchen for days afterward!

8. **Use the garbage pail.** Better to throw away fat- and calorie-laden foods than your self-esteem, self-confidence, hard work, and skinny jeans. Are you still having a hard time parting with pretzels because you feel guilty about wasting food? Here's a thought: donate the food to a local shelter or religious institution, both of which provide daily meals for the less fortunate. You'll feel much better, even relieved, to have the tempting food out of reach.

9. **Don't forget to eat during the day before the event.** Skipping meals is probably the biggest no-no for dieters. Going more than three to four hours without eating sends your body into deprivation mode and may trigger binge-eating. Have a salad, low-calorie soup, or some fruit before you start feeling hungry.

10. **Put a selection of light foods on display.** Other guests are sure to be grateful to have some healthy selections.

11. **Learn to share.** Did someone bring truffles or your favorite peanut brittle as a hostess gift? Take them with you to your next party or to work, or give them away as gifts to people who make your life a little easier or happier. (Regifting is okay here!) You want to share the joy . . . and calories!

If You're the Guest . . .

1. **Ask the host what he or she will be serving.** This way, you can formulate a same-day food plan that will set you up for success at the event.

2. **Get physical earlier in the day.** When you're the host, you run around getting the house and everything else ready for company. If you're an invitee, you get to have the day off! Try to fit in a walk, hit the gym, or play the exercise video you've been meaning to try.

3. **Be sneaky.** Carry your own salad dressing packets or low-calorie alternative chocolate bar in your bag. Use them to help you say no to hidden calories or certain foods without feeling like you're missing out. I often eat my Chocolite Bar on the car ride home!

4. **Offer to bring a dish.** Check in with the host ahead of time and find out what you can contribute. Then bring

a good guy alternative. Your host will love the help, and you'll know you're covered.

5. **Take a 30-minute time-out.** Wait until you've been at the party for at least 30 minutes until you start eating. This gives you time to relax when you first walk in, get involved in the festivities, and survey the best food picks for your diet plan.

6. **Use smaller plates.** A salad plate for a dinner buffet, for example. Fill half with fruit or vegetables.

Either Way . . .

1. **Don't fast all day or go hungry to the party.** Being around all new foods will cause you to eat with your eyes, not your belly. Take the edge off your hunger before the party. Have a vegetable soup or large salad.

2. **Have a substantial breakfast.** And a light lunch. Drink a lot of zero-calorie beverages and have high-protein, high-fiber snacks. Don't do the "I'm saving up for the big meal" thing. It's a bad idea. If you're hungry and thirsty at the big meal, you'll probably overeat.

3. **Watch the alcohol—those calories add up.** If you drink a lot of alcohol, you're more likely to make poor food decisions because of your blurry head.

4. **Always carry a low-calorie drink in your dominant hand at parties.** Put tomato juice, diet soda, or a wine spritzer in a wineglass to treat it as a special drink. This keeps your hand and mouth busy so you have less involvement with the food.

5. **Eat with your nondominant hand.** If you're a righty, use your left hand to eat appetizers, or vice versa. It's harder and more awkward to eat with your nondominant hand, so it slows you down and makes you pay better attention to how much food you're eating.

6. **At cocktail parties, devote yourself to low-calorie staples.** Crudité, shrimp, and grilled kebabs are best bets.

7. **Move away from the buffet.** We eat with our eyes, so never stand near the buffet table! Take one or two items, then move away.

8. **Take a plate (or cocktail napkin).** Always eat off of a plate. Don't graze all night. You won't register what you ate. Fill a plate and have your meal or appetizers.

9. **Say no to communal eating.** We eat more when we eat from a group dish. Think family style, chip bowls, sushi platters, and so on. Taking your own plate will slow you down. You'll pay attention and probably eat less.

10. **Cruise and then commit.** If you want to try a sampling of the different foods offered, cruise first, then commit to filling your plate with lean meat and vegetables, saving room for one or two splurges.

11. **Follow the half-plate rule.** Half the plate should be vegetables (valuable real estate here!) and the other half should be the two or three items you really want to eat. The key is to remember that you're having only one plate of food.

12. **If you think the first taste of a particular food could set off a binge, don't take that first bite.** It may be easier than trying to stop after the taste is in your mouth.

13. **Use calorie-saving tips.** Eat the filling of a pie or quiche, not the crust. Fill your plate with vegetables and then take a spoonful of pasta or rice.

14. **Use smaller plates.** A salad plate for a dinner buffet, for example.

15. **Start and end your meal with a hot soup or beverage.** Sipping on broth-based soups before a meal will help fill you up, and having some tea or coffee at the end of a meal (I also love hot water with lemon and a packet of zero-calorie sweetener) will keep your hands and mouth busy so it's easier to say no to high-calorie desserts.

Living with Others: A House Full of Food

PART OF LIVING IN THE REAL WORLD IS LIVING WITH OTHER PEOPLE and their food preferences. Unfortunately, their food choices don't always agree with ours. I often hear clients say, "I need to keep those foods around for my kids," or, "I can't punish my family because I'm on a diet." While this is compelling reasoning, it's just not true. You can set some boundaries in your own home, making bad boyfriend foods something to only be eaten outside the house and not feeling guilty if family members don't have 24-hour access to them.

That being said, I am realistic—you have to pick your battles. Here are some strategies to help you live with others in a house of food:

1. **Go opaque and save.** Our favorite foods usually come in cute, tempting, inviting packages. Advertisers know that the package alone can draw us in, even before we open it! Take your tempting foods out of the product box/container/bag and put them into opaque containers or Ziploc bags. Some of the appeal will instantly diminish.

2. **Measure, measure, measure!** Get measuring bowls, cups, and spoons that are already portioned. It will save you a step, calories, and lots of guesswork. To make portion control a little more fun, go to portionware.com for bowls in pretty colors. Remember to use the largest bowl for your veggies!

3. **Get your bad boyfriends out and your good guys in!** Replace your trigger foods with foods that you have control around and that help with your weight loss.

4. **Declutter.** If there are foods in your pantry, fridge, or freezer that you haven't touched in six months (yuck!), toss them. Clutter is distracting: it can make you lose sight of your food goals and take away from the foods you want to be eating.

5. **Hide, but don't seek.** Store bad boyfriend foods brought in for family members out of sight. Keep them off of counters where they are in full view. Put them in the back of the fridge. Place those good guys front and center!

6. **Show off your good guys.** Display fruits and veggies and other good guys on the counter in that pretty bowl you love. Put them in clear containers in the fridge so they catch your eye right away.

7. **Stock up on stuff you don't like.** If you're not a fan of raisins, buy oatmeal-raisin cookies for the kids' lunches. Don't use those cute kids as an excuse to treat yourself to your favorites!

8. **Use an oil sprayer.** Olive oil is full of monounsaturated fats and antioxidants, making it a heart-healthy power food. But whether you bought it in Naples or your local supermarket, it costs you 120 calories per tablespoon. Douse your broccoli with a quick "splash" of olive oil and you can easily add three tablespoons of oil, which translates into 360 calories! Use zero-calorie olive oil cooking spray or an oil mist sprayer directly on your food.

Although not every spray is entirely calorie-free (any food with five calories or less per serving can make a calorie-free claim), it's a lot better than spooning or drizzling oil on your food, calorically speaking.

9. **Ban the clean plate club.** The clean plate club is all well and good if you're washing dishes—but only then. If your son leaves three bites of pizza on his plate and it ends up in your mouth, congratulations—you've just consumed 100 mindless calories. If he's old enough, have him scrape his plate into the garbage so you won't be the human garbage pail. Otherwise, be diligent and get it into the garbage yourself. Better there than on your thighs!

GIRLS' NIGHT OUT

Birthdays. Mah-jongg. Book club. Ever go out with the girls and find yourself digging into the chips and guacamole or the family-style penne vodka faster than Fred Flintstone said "Yabba-dabba-doo"? While we love each other's company, being with a group of women can take its toll on the best-laid diet plans. Here are some strategies for your favorite girls' night out.

1. **Be a trendsetter!** A new study found that women eating in groups mimic each other's eating behaviors and mannerisms. So if a friend reaches for that

chocolate chip cookie, it increases the chances that you will too. Don't get new friends—lead the pack! Reach for low-calorie alternatives, bring a healthy dish, or order wisely—and watch as others follow your lead.

2. **Order a salad or broth-based soup.** When the girls order fried calamari (or some other non-diet-friendly appetizer) for the group, you can order a low-calorie alternative at the same time. You want to be busy eating—and avoid reaching for that loaded nacho chip.

3. **Eat from your own plate.** Eating in a large group can instill a subconscious fear that if you don't get in there quickly, the food will disappear. My client Heather loves to go out for sushi to celebrate just about anything. To avoid overeating, she now asks for a small plate, chooses five pieces of her favorite sushi (see page 138), and keeps them all to herself. At our next session, Heather told me that she'd felt calmer, eaten more slowly, and enjoyed the company more than ever.

4. **Have fun!** Chances are you've tasted every food you've ever wanted. Focus on the company and the atmosphere. Don't live to eat . . . eat to live! Then just do it!

Frozen Yogurt: Friend or Foe?

MANY OF MY CLIENTS REPORT THAT THEIR FAVORITE THING TO do on weekends is to hit a frozen yogurt shop, get a small nonfat cup with one fruit topping, and savor it as if it were the hottest summer's day. Self-serve frozen yogurt places are on every street corner these days! They are especially popular with kids. But most kids are not as worried as It Girls are about piling on the calories and fat. So here's what to look out for if you decide to venture into your nearest frozen yogurt shop:

1. **Oversize cups.** Fro-yo chains are marketing mavens. They give you huge cups so you'll fill them to the brim without blinking an eye. We tend to help ourselves to double the listed serving size (usually a half-cup).

2. **The scale.** Not the bathroom scale—the store's checkout scale. Since it's easy to fill 'er up (see number 1), fill your cup a little bit, then go weigh it. Continue to do this until you get the serving size you want based on the calories you want to consume. Don't worry if the cashiers glare at you. Trust me, they've seen it before.

3. **Your flavor.** Some yogurt shops offer many different flavors on any given day. This means the eight-calorie-per-ounce option may be right next to the twenty-calorie-per-ounce option. It can be fun to mix a few flavors, but don't overlook the different calorie counts as you do so.

4. **Toppings.** They add up *fast*. It doesn't matter if your frozen yogurt has only eight calories an ounce and you took four ounces. If you load up with chocolate pieces and nuts, you can add tons of calories by the time you're done.

   - *Top first.* Instead of putting your toppings on last, put them on first. Scoop out some mini marshmallows (just two calories each) or a teaspoon of sprinkles (twenty calories) or some fresh fruit. Then add your four ounces of frozen yogurt over it. You'll end up taking fewer toppings if you use this reverse-order trick.

   - *Trick toppers.* You know candy, fudge, and caramel are not diet-friendly choices. But some toppings that *look* innocent are anything but. Steer clear of fruit in sugary syrup (choose fresh fruit instead), sugar-free syrups and fudge toppings (they still have tons of fat and calories), fat-free gummy candy (the calories from sugar pack a punch), and crushed nuts and granola (a quarter-cup adds 100 calories!).

5. **Be on the lookout for cones.** While a sugar cone has 50 calories and a wafer cone 20 calories, it's often a good choice to use a cone for forced portion control. Only about four ounces can fit in the cone, and there are also limits on how much topping can adhere to the treat.

It's Five O'Clock Somewhere!
The Dos and Don'ts of Skinny Jeans Drinking

ALCOHOL IS THE ULTIMATE SIMPLE CARBOHYDRATE. SIMPLY PUT, it contains nothing except a pile of empty calories. But dieting is for the long haul—and as noted, you've got to have fun. So I've concocted some rules to observe for imbibing on any occasion:

1. **Do opt for a glass of wine or light beer.** A 12-ounce bottle of light beer has around 100 calories, and a 5-ounce glass of wine has about 120 calories.

   - If you encounter a bartender with a heavy wine pour (over 5 ounces), go for either champagne served in a smaller champagne flute (90 calories) or a wine spritzer (120 calories per 12 ounces).

   - If you're at home, measure out 5 ounces before putting it in your usual glass. You can then eyeball the right portion.

   - *Note on wine calories:* While a 5-ounce glass of wine per day at 120 calories may seem harmless, that will add up to an extra 1,700 calories over two and a half weeks. That is the equivalent of about half a pound of body fat on the scale—and your hips.

2. **Don't start with the bar bites.** Those items are fried, fatty, salty, carb-heavy, and dirty (think of all the hands that were in them). So don't skip dinner in an effort to save your calories for alcohol. If you do, you're more likely to be tempted by those high-calorie snacks. Have a light meal

before going out drinking, and look for some light noshes during the happy hour, such as shrimp cocktail, chicken skewers, or a raw bar.

3. **Don't be color-blind.** Stick to clear or light-colored alcohol with 100 calories per 1.5-ounce shot. Vodka, rum, and tequila are great choices. Don't forget the flavored varieties to add some extra zip. A one-shot drink over ice with a calorie-free mixer such as diet tonic, diet soda, or light juice is a great, light way to drink.

4. **Do watch out for those mixers.** Club soda has no calories, and tonic water has 80 calories per cup. How ironic! Choose diet tonic or diet soda as your zero-calorie mixers. Sugar-free powdered drink mixes also taste refreshing.

5. **Do take a splash, not a soaking.** Fruit juices contain lots of calories. A splash for flavor is okay, but half a cup will add 60 calories to your drink.

6. **Do be social.** The more time you spend talking and dancing, the less time you're eating and drinking. For a smart dance move, boogie your booty away from the bar.

You can keep control of your diet, no matter where you eat or drink. Just because you're going to eat out doesn't mean all bets are off. Simply keep this chapter flagged so you can order smart, stay on track, and be ready for any dining situation that comes your way!

CHAPTER 8

Maintenance: Living and Thriving in the World of Food

SINCE SHE STARTED DIETING AT THE TENDER AGE OF 15, Claudia has lost, by her own estimation, nearly 900 pounds.

Three years ago, she wanted to shed some weight for her 25th college reunion. Last year she wanted to look good at her daughter's high school graduation. When she hit 40, her doctor told her that losing weight would help lower her cholesterol and blood pressure. Just a month ago, she needed a new wardrobe but didn't want to be seen scouring the plus-size racks at the local department store.

Each time Claudia starts a diet, she has the best of intentions. She's super-motivated, always has a goal in mind, and will do anything to achieve it. Calorie restriction, juice fasting, skipping meals, fruits and veggies only—the method is always secondary to the goal of losing weight. By any objective measure, Claudia is a successful dieter. But here's one thing I neglected to mention: in the 35 years since she first started dieting, Claudia has gained more than 1,000 pounds. In the world of dieting, Claudia has maxed out her credit cards. She's forever overspending—and always in the red!

For Claudia, success on the scale has proved elusive. No matter what diet she tries, sooner or later she returns to her old ways and the pounds come back—often with a few friends in tow. Claudia's problem isn't uncommon. In fact, the most daunting challenge facing dieters isn't weight loss. Nearly all dieters lose some weight no matter what program they follow. The problem is that most dieters don't know how to keep the weight off.

Here's a startling statistic: every year 45 million people in this country start a diet. There are now 75 million active dieters in the United States. Within a year, 66 percent of those 75 million will gain back one-third of the weight they lose, and 97 percent will gain it all back in just five years. The problem isn't losing weight. Almost every dieter loses some weight. The problem is keeping it off.

Why Can't We Keep It Off?

IN RECENT YEARS, RESEARCH HAS FOCUSED ON UNLOCKING THE complex biological processes that might help explain why dieters have little trouble losing weight but struggle to keep it off. Some have reasoned that our calorie-craving bodies effectively sabotage our attempts at weight loss, holding on to those precious calories to avoid the starvation that afflicted our earliest ancestors. Others have speculated that after many years of being overweight, our bodies adapt, altering the way we regulate weight by stimulating our appetite to protect their precious fat stores. Metabolism shifts as well once we lose weight. A newly thin body needs 8 to 10 fewer calories per day for each pound of weight that's been lost. A gal who loses 30 pounds requires about 240 to 300 fewer calories each day than she did before the weight started disappearing. And don't forget your hormones; they can play havoc with your weight and waistline. Some studies show that after a weight loss, levels of the appetite-regulating hormone leptin drop, making it harder for us to control our cravings, especially for our favorite bad boyfriend foods.

These are interesting findings, and from a strictly scientific point of view they make perfect sense. But what the scientists are missing is the uniquely human element of weight loss. Dieting is a pain-motivated behavior. No one goes on a diet because they're happy. They're in pain—about being ridiculed, about feeling worthless and ashamed, about feeling out of control, and about not fitting into their favorite clothes. Since the pain of being overweight can be almost unbearable, most dieters will do anything to get thin. I see 30 clients a week on average, and I can say that almost all come into my office because they're in this kind of pain and will do anything to get rid of it.

But once the weight comes off and the pain passes, they forget. They start canceling appointments, they stop following my tricks and tips, and they don't think about their bad boyfriend foods. This is normal. Our minds are designed to move us past the memories of unpleasant experiences. However, when we lose our vigilance, we gain the weight back. This is the biggest problem for dieters.

Dieters are repeat offenders. Like I said, no one starts a diet because they're happy. They're unhappy with the way they look in clothes or the way they feel getting dressed. They're tired of staying home on a Saturday night or having no energy to run after their kids. They just can't enjoy this way of living anymore. Is the pain of being fat, unhappy, insecure, and uncomfortable enough pain for you?

The Big Booby Prize

WHEN I STARTED LOSING WEIGHT, I THOUGHT I'D FINALLY START living the life I'd dreamed of. I had a goal in mind and I was super-motivated. I began every day with the following thought: *When I'm thin I'll. . . .* I'd spent the better part of two decades pinning my hopes, dreams, and expectations on the back of being skinny, and now I was on the way to reaching my lifelong goal of being thin. But a funny thing happened when I finally got thin. I quickly realized that getting to the top of the mountain wasn't nearly as difficult as staying there.

After I lost weight and started fitting into a smaller size of clothing, I thought: *Game over. I've arrived.* This was the new, thin Lyssa, and she wasn't going anywhere. I could do or eat anything I wanted. I was calling the shots and finally felt in control in my life.

I was wrong. Though I'd lost weight, I hadn't lost the problem. I was still thinking like a fat girl. The weight was gone, the scale had dropped, and my dress size had shrunk, but my head was still the same. Within three months of stopping my diet I'd gained back nearly all the weight I'd lost.

My story isn't uncommon. Every day millions of dieters in this country lose weight. But nearly all of them gain it back—often with interest. This is why I tell my clients that losing weight is a big booby prize. People who lose weight think they've crossed the finish line. But losing weight isn't like running a 10K race. There may be a finish line to weight loss, but there's no finish line to weight management. It's an ongoing, lifelong process.

Forget the Weight, Focus on the Process

MOST DIETERS MAKE THE MISTAKE I MADE. THEY HAVE A GOAL weight, and once they reach it they think, *That's it.* But getting thin is one thing; staying thin is another matter altogether. Anyone can lose weight, but few people can keep it off. Why is that? Most dieters don't realize that the *process of staying thin*—not getting thin—is the goal.

Scores of diet books and weight loss programs ask the same (wrong) question: "What's your target weight?" The right question should be: "How do you plan to change your thinking?" Weight is just a symptom—a symptom of being out of control with food. If you don't change your thinking, you'll never truly reach your goal. And the goal is staying thin.

Rethinking Thin

HAVE YOU EVER THOUGHT ABOUT WHAT IT MEANS TO LOSE WEIGHT? Does it mean changing your dress size? Does it mean losing a few pounds? Does it mean having a richer social life or feeling more attractive?

If you answered "yes" to any of these questions, you'd be dead wrong. What does fitting into a smaller size of clothing mean if you're still tormented daily by a piece of cake, a bread basket, or a chocolate chip cookie? What does seeing the scale drop mean if you're still haunted by self-loathing, guilt, shame, and feelings of failure? The millions who lose weight but still struggle to live comfortably in the world of food are no better off than the alcoholic who struggles to live comfortably sober. There's nothing that compares to the peace of mind that comes from knowing that you're finally in control of food.

Like an addict who has just left rehab, a dieter needs to know that the time right after weight loss is the most dangerous time. Many dieters think that since they've lost weight, they're "cured" and will never be fat again. But as soon as they relax their vigilance, the pounds come back. This kind of thing happens again and again, whether it's the first time or the twentieth. I can't tell you how many clients come back to my office mystified that they're fat again. "I was really good," they say. "I don't know how this happened."

I tell them, as I tell anyone who struggles with their weight, that they've let go of the very things that helped them get thin in the first place.

Part of the problem is the nature of dieting itself. Dieting is a concrete, structured way of eating. People who are out of control with food need to be reined in and need clearly defined boundaries. They need to be told what they can and can't eat. They need a food routine with regularly scheduled meals and snacks.

But once the weight comes off and the diet is lifted, everything falls apart. The structure and organization that helped them control their eating is gone. These dieters head back into the world of food with just a few admonitions to eat sensibly. Hello? Most dieters can't eat sensibly. If they could, they wouldn't have started dieting in the first place! It takes more than an admonition to eat sensibly and control behavior that's been out of control for decades.

Vigilance: Your Best Tool

HAVE YOU EVER BEEN TO AN ALCOHOLICS ANONYMOUS MEETING? Someone raises a hand and says, "Hi, I'm Dan, and I'm an alcoholic. I've been 20 years sober." You might have thought, *Why is Dan still coming to meetings if he's been sober for 20 years?*

Here's a news flash. Dan has maintained his sobriety for 20 years because he still goes to meetings. The meetings, where he shares with other alcoholics and has the opportunity to mentor and sponsor, have provided Dan with a valuable tool: vigilance. Dan has stayed sober for 20 years because he knows that he's an addict and always will be. Physical addiction to alcohol may end after rehab, but recovery is a lifelong process.

In this way, dieters are just like alcoholics. The compulsion to abuse food is always there. It's ingrained in the subconscious of most dieters. I've maintained my weight loss for nearly 20 years, but I know that at any moment I could fall off the wagon and quickly return to my old patterns. It's only by staying vigilant that I stay thin. I'll admit I've struggled at times. Returning to work, financial pressures, family illness, consecutive snow days—all these things have tested my resolve. That's why it is so important to stay on top of things.

I like to joke with my clients that we're always in remission. We can't lose sight of where we started. The thinking that got us into trouble in the first place doesn't go away when we change our weight or clothing size.

Doing Away with "All Foods in Moderation"

FEW THINGS HAVE DONE MORE TO DERAIL THE AMBITIONS OF DIET-ers than the popular advice to enjoy all foods in moderation. The problem with this otherwise well-intentioned advice is that it doesn't account for the fact that if we could eat moderately we wouldn't have needed to diet in the first place.

Nearly every diet program ever created encourages its clients to eat moderately, as though they're leery of telling them that any food is off limits. One popular weight loss program assigns points to promote all foods in moderation, both during the weight loss phase and on maintenance. Once you lift the structure of the diet and start thinking you can have some of your bad boys in moderation, you're at risk of gaining back your weight. You didn't change your thinking.

The message isn't getting through to millions of dieters, and that's why so many gain back the weight they worked so hard to lose. The message can't be "all foods in moderation." That might work for the 3 percent of It Girls, but it doesn't work for you. You have to maintain structure, support, the framework, and your personal strategies. A diet only lasts for so long, but you want thin to last into your fifties, sixties, and even seventies!

The Keys to Successful Maintenance

1. **Find a good guy you're crazy about.** After all, you're not a martyr. Find something you enjoy. *Really* enjoy. (Make it worthwhile!) If you love a good chocolate bar (typically 250 calories), try a Chocolite chocolate bar for 95 calories. Flip back to the list of good guy alternatives (page 226) and use it liberally!

2. **Breaking up is hard to do.** "Breaking up is like knocking over a Coke machine. You can't do it in one push," Jerry Seinfeld famously said. The same thing applies to breaking up with bad boyfriend foods. Even if you swear off baked goods, you may find yourself absentmindedly nibbling on animal crackers as you prepare your son's lunchbox for

the next day (speaking from experience here). Perfection is impossible—and it's also a matter of opinion. Slipups occur and are totally normal, so please don't beat yourself up. Most of all, stop quickly. Living thin is a skill, and it takes a lot of practice. Just be aware when you've slipped up, forgive yourself, stay focused, and get back on track.

Unfortunately, we're so good at beating ourselves up that forgiving ourselves doesn't come easily. When we think we've blown it, we give up and go on a rampage. When this happens, please change your internal dialogue—tell yourself you *will* do better next time. Tell yourself that mistakes will happen. Tell yourself you're worth fighting for.

Personal note: As a thin person, I'm able to recover from a slipup much more quickly. That's not just a reason to pat myself on the back—my ability to make a quick recovery potentially subtracts hundreds or even thousands of calories from my hips and keeps the scale in check! Now I say, "Lyssa, you ate half of the bag of baked chips. It's okay. Just stop now. Put the bag away and back slowly out of the kitchen." Then I brush my teeth, chew a piece of gum, or turn on the TV. I've pulled myself back from the edge so many times now that I know I'll be just fine.

3. **Don't "repent."** Don't try to make up for your slipup by starving yourself or going on an exercise binge. Remember the rules on emotional eating from page 85: you *will* either get hungry (and binge) or feel deprived (and binge). Simply refrain from looking back—the past is the past, period.

Personal note: I recall potty training my son, which was

grueling. I never screamed and yelled (well, I did, but in the bathroom when he wasn't looking, or on the phone to my husband, who seemed to suddenly have a lot of late meetings). I never told my son he was a failure or would be in diapers forever. Instead of yelling, I coached him—told him he could do it, that it wasn't easy but he'd figure it out. I came at his accidents with love and support and encouragement. We give it to our children. We should give it to ourselves too.

4. **Keep a temptation-free kitchen.** Keep all bad boyfriend foods out of your house, where emotional eating is most prevalent. Eat your bad boyfriend foods only in controlled situations, such as Raisinets at the movies (and be sure to share the box). Even a low-calorie food can be a bad boy if you eat too much of it or eat it in an out-of-control way. Evaluate a food based, not on the calories it represents, but on your behavior around it.

My client Julie opens a bag of white cheddar rice cakes and the whole bag instantly disappears. It may not be chocolate éclairs, but nevertheless it's her bad boy food. Another example is nuts—specifically, almonds. I should have the marketing team that almonds have! We have been told by so many different sources—advertisements, cardiologists, vegans—that almonds are some kind of miracle food, high in protein, with monounsaturated (heart-healthy) fat and antioxidants. But 20 almonds contain 160 calories. They're easy to down, and they're fatty and often salty. So if you have a thing for almonds, they're a problem. This doesn't mean you should never eat almonds, but bringing them into your home environment may be a bad idea. Having a handful at a friend's house or over a salad may be a smarter move. It's not just about calories—it's also about control.

5. **Weigh yourself either daily or every other day.** Try to do it at the same time each day, and in the same clothes. This way you stay accountable, keep track of your progress, and avoid slipping into denial if you backslide. If you ate a salty meal, are ovulating, or are about to get your period, your weight will almost surely go up by three or four pounds. Don't panic: it's just water weight. It will work its way out of your body in a day or two.

    Allow yourself a four-pound weight variation, and no more. If you see the scale increase more than that, it's time to go back to your diet and the strategies that worked for you in the weight loss phase.

6. **Watch those *bites, licks, and tastes (BLTs)*.** BLTs can add up to real calories and make all the difference between weight loss, weight maintenance, and weight gain. I like to think of every bite, lick, and taste as a 25-calorie unit. If 150 extra calories a day is all it takes to put on 15 pounds in a year, that means 150 less calories a day is what it takes to take it off. Go back and reread chapter 2.

7. **If you bite it, write it.** Relatedly, keep your food log at all times, or record what you eat on your computer, iPad, smartphone, or a scrap of paper. A food journal works as

an effective tool only if you use it—particularly if you feel your weight creeping back up. Here are some tips on making a food record work for you:

- *Get a journal you can travel with.* If it's too big, you'll leave it at home. The purpose is to write as you go, so the journal needs to be with you at all times. Some clients ask me if they can keep a record of what they are eating in an app. I often recommend MyFitnessPal or Lose It!, but some of my clients, even those who are tech-savvy, still prefer to track their food the old-fashioned way and write it down. Really, whatever works for you.

- *Be prompt. Do* write as you eat; otherwise, you'll forget exactly what you ate and how much. Don't wait until evening and try to remember. Invariably you'll forget a little snack or treat. You may also underestimate your portion sizes.

- *Measure and record portion sizes as best as you can.*

- *Tell the truth.* You may be tempted to gloss over some of your food choices. While you may feel guilt or shame, don't do this. If you are honest, you can take a hard look at your patterns and emotional triggers and recognize them the next time you are faced with a similar food choice or situation.

- *Make notes.* Take note of the circumstances or feelings that led to a slipup. These sidebar notes can enlighten you as to how to avoid the next one.

- *Record your weight and daily goals.* A goal can be as simple as the ability to climb into bed and say, "Today was a good eating day."

- *Don't forget your drinks.* Calories from drinks count! That skinny latte or low-sugar cranberry juice goes toward your overall intake. Also, they can undermine the effort to drink more water and to cut down on diet soda or wine.

- *Be grateful.* Oprah popularized the "gratitude journal." If you want to focus on positive emotions, write three things a day in your food journal that you are grateful for or happy about. Focusing on the positive makes us feel happier, which leads to less comfort food and better decisions overall.

- *Review often.* A food journal isn't helpful if you don't review the information you've written down. Designate a time each week to sit down and go over your food journal information. I look mine over on Sunday nights. It helps me think about what my week was like, notice patterns, and plan my goals for the upcoming week.

8. **Set goals and give rewards.** Goals keep you moving forward, and rewards keep you motivated. Buy yourself a new lipstick for running that 5K. Sleep in on Saturday for maintaining your weight all week. Cook yourself a nice, light gourmet meal as a reward for avoiding the Häagen-Dazs your husband put in the freezer.

9. **Follow the three-bite rule.** If you do want to taste something that's not on your maintenance plan, just have three bites of it. Our taste buds are the most aware, or

sensitized, for the first three bites of a food. After that, we don't taste the food as fully.

10. **Go for 50 percent vegetables.** This strategy is similar to my half-plate rule. Fifty percent of your calories at lunch and dinner should come from vegetables. Veggies are the volumizer in your maintenance food plan and will keep you fuller, longer.

VEGETABLES: PRIME PLATE REAL ESTATE

While you're maintaining your weight, make sure vegetables take up the most real estate on the plate. Barbara Rolls, chair of the Nutritional Sciences Department at Penn State University, pooled all the data on more than 700 people in the Premier trial, a study that showed people can feel fuller by eating low-density foods, and found that an increase in vegetables is a reliable predictor of whether people have lost weight—and how much they lost. By eating a diet high in vegetables, people can fill themselves up, but for fewer calories. And it works!

Studies that look at consistent weight loss maintainers—people who have lost at least 10 percent of their maximum body weight and maintained the loss for at least five years—find that maintainers eat three to five times more vegetables than people who are overweight or normal weight. We're talking about the elite 3 percent of girls here. It's the secret to their success at winning at weight loss.

PART TWO

The Skinny Jeans Diet

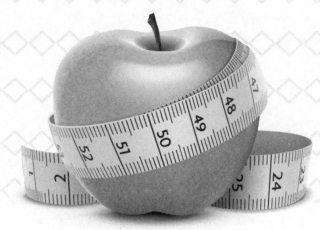

S INCE THE SKINNY JEANS DIET IS A THINKING PLAN AND NOT just an eating plan, the foods, recipes, shopping lists, and guidelines provided in this part of the book don't arbitrarily follow some government-designed healthy "food pyramid" or "food plate." Rather, they follow your unique relationship with food. Remember, there's no such thing as a good eating plan that doesn't consider the most important variable in weight management—you!

The Skinny Jeans Diet is simple and easy to follow. All of the foods and the recipe ingredients are available at supermarket chains, gourmet food shops, and health food stores, or you can order them online through retailers like Whole Foods, Peapod, and Fresh Direct. The diet's synergistic 50/30/20 meals and recipes (carbohydrates/proteins/fats) promote satiety, curb cravings, and provide great nutrition while keeping excess calories in check. This eating plan avoids the rigid guidelines and strict rules that cause so many dieters to get frustrated and throw in the towel. Instead, the Skinny Jeans Diet provides a framework upon which you can design a way of eating that fits your own preferences, habits, personality, lifestyle, and relationship with food.

Phase I, the Skinny Jeans Three-Day Detox, is designed to jump-start your metabolism. It's filled with the very best foods for safe, rapid weight loss. This is the most structured phase of the diet, since it's important to rein in and organize behavior that's been out of control. Hence, I've avoided giving you too many choices in this phase of the diet. Thank God it's only for three days! Remember also that variety stimulates consumption, and too many options may cause you to feel overwhelmed.

Phase II, the Master Weight Loss Plan, is different from Phase I in that you stay on it until you hit your target weight. During this phase, weight loss slows a little. That's intentional. If you lose too much weight too quickly, your thyroid gland, which regulates your metabolism, kicks into starvation mode and you end up burning fewer calories. I tell my clients that while you may be excited to fit into that little red bikini, your body has its own agenda. It's only interested in protecting your vital organs and providing enough fuel to sustain the activities of daily living. The other reason weight loss slows during this phase is that more variety is offered. More than anything, this phase of the diet is about peace of mind. As one client told me recently, "It is the most amazing feeling to wake up and my first thought is not about food or how I'm going to eat today. I have a rhythm and routine with eating that I feel good about. My mind is free for other things."

Once you get within three pounds of your target weight, it's time to think about shifting from the Master Weight Loss Plan to Phase III—Maintenance. Since this is an eating plan for life, Phase III offers the greatest variety of foods. Yet you're not at risk now of gaining back what you lost because there's a difference of only 100 to 200 calories between the weight loss and weight maintenance phases of this diet. My clients often ask, "Lyssa, I've reached my goal. What should I be eating now?" My answer always is the same: "What you did and ate to lose weight is what you will do and eat to maintain that loss." As Brenda Wolfe, Ph.D., founder and clinical director of the esteemed Eating Disorders Institute of New Mexico, writes in *Weight Control Digest*, "The first essential step in preventing relapse is eliminating the artificial boundary between weight loss and weight maintenance."

What Makes This a Great Diet?

MORE THAN JUST A BIOLOGICAL FUNCTION, EATING IS ONE OF LIFE'S greatest pleasures, and food and drink are woven into our social fabric. From birth to death, nearly every social occasion is accompanied by a meal, snack, or something to drink. We toast our best friend's wedding. A Jewish child's bat mitzvah always is followed with a meal. Global Village Day at your daughter's school centers on the experience of sampling food from other cultures. In Thailand, it's customary to collect several dozen favorite recipes in a booklet to be distributed at your funeral. In Japan, pleasure is promoted as a goal of healthy eating. "Make all activities pertaining to food and eating pleasurable ones," says a widely disseminated Japanese government guideline. Norway offers similar advice to its citizens: "*Food* + Joy + Health." And Great Britain and Korea suggest, "Enjoy your food." Clearly, food is a defining feature of a full life.

The Skinny Jeans Diet acknowledges that for the majority of people, eating goes far beyond nutrition. But in a country where almost 70 percent of the adult population is overweight or obese, how do we reconcile the obvious conflict between enjoying the many delicious things the world has to offer and wanting to obtain and maintain a slender waistline? For starters, you need to choose an eating plan that does the following:

1. Recognizes and honors your past troubled relationship with certain bad boyfriend foods
2. Provides safe and steady weight loss
3. Leaves you feeling satisfied without feeling too full
4. Gives you the biggest bang for your buck, allowing you to fill your plate without tipping the scale
5. Offers structure but doesn't overwhelm with rules and restrictions
6. Helps you look and feel like a million bucks
7. Is easy to follow and fits into your day-to-day lifestyle
8. Offers many alternatives to the bad boyfriend foods you love
9. And, let's not forget, helps you fit into your skinny jeans

The Skinny Jeans Diet is loaded from top to bottom with foods that fit neatly within the tricks, tips, and guidelines offered in the pages of this book. It avoids the high-calorie, high-fat foods that are at the root of most people's weight problems and replaces them with a rich assortment of delicious light foods, which many of my clients, including the most obdurate food addicts, seem to prefer over their higher-calorie counterparts. Hence, this section includes multiple lists of great-tasting, low-fat, and low-calorie alternatives to our favorite bad boyfriend foods. Check out the resources found on page 226 for a comprehensive list of the names and contact information of many of the recommended brands.

I'll also offers guidelines in this section for dealing with common food situations, suggestions for the very best foods for quick but healthy weight loss, and advice for what to do once you've hit your weight loss goals so you don't get bored.

Personalize It!

THERE IS NO SINGLE DIET THAT'S PERFECT FOR EVERYONE. EACH OF us brings our own unique behavior, personality, and preferences to the table. One person's trash is another person's treasure. Or as we say in the Skinny Jeans Diet world, one's girl's frock is another girl's gorgeous couture gown.

For any eating plan to be the right plan for you, it has to be personalized. Though I offer suggestions for the best times to schedule meals and snacks, these are by no means written in cement. I have one client who loves her midafternoon snack but can't eat anything after seven or eight o'clock at night, since eating too late keeps her up. On the other hand, I also have a client who can't turn in and go to bed without having something to eat. One client, the mother of four children, all under the age of eight, needs to squeeze in her meals and snacks around school schedules and after-school activities. Whatever you decide, the eating plan must work with the realities of your day-to-day life.

GO PUBLIC

Tell your goals to a friend, family member, or even the taxi driver. This helps you to be accountable. You can also phone a friend or get a weight loss buddy. Weight loss (and weight gain) can be contagious (like poison ivy, but not as itchy). Studies show that women lose an average of 10 pounds more than they otherwise would when they diet and exercise together. Having a buddy gives you an immediate support system, and sharing the journey makes sticking to commitments easier and more fun when your motivation begins to fade.

Go Lean and Green

IT'S OFTEN SAID BUT CAN'T BE REPEATED ENOUGH: YOUR DIET should include a generous amount of dark green, leafy vegetables and lean protein. Vegetables in particular are a high-volume food, meaning that they contain a lot of water and fiber. As a result, they're filling but don't cost you a lot of calories. High-volume foods help fill you up and leave you satisfied. Ideally, and with some exceptions such as white potatoes and butternut squash, vegetables should make up 50 percent of your lunch and dinner calories. Here's the best part: on the Skinny Jeans Diet, vegetables, provided they're not smothered in butter or oil, are free!

Lean protein also gives high volume per calorie. Did you know that you could have six ounces of steamed or boiled shrimp for just 200 calories? Or that you could dive into a two-pound lobster for just 228 calories? (As long as you avoid the melted butter!) If you don't like seafood or fish, try white meat poultry, egg whites, low-fat cheese and yogurt, or a meatless protein source like tofu. Many popular veggies are rich in protein as well, including asparagus, broccoli, artichokes, and sweet corn. I tell my clients that when their weight loss plateaus, they can give it a quick kick in the pants by eating more lean protein and green, nonstarchy veggies.

Should You Avoid Packaged, Processed Foods?

It's sad but very true: a majority of Americans have been carrying on a torrid affair with processed and packaged foods. As a nifty little article in the *New York Times* points out, "Americans eat 31 percent more packaged food than fresh food, and they consume more packaged food per person than their counterparts in nearly all other countries. A sizable part of the American diet is ready-to-eat meals, like frozen pizzas and microwave dinners, and sweet or salty snack foods."

This shouldn't come as much of a shock. Processed and packaged foods are affordable and convenient, fitting easily into our wallets and hectic lifestyles. And let's be frank: they often taste great. The real problem with processed, packaged food is that a majority of the choices are high in calories, low in nutrition, and loaded with sugar, fat, and salt. Many of my clients complain that processed foods don't satisfy their hunger. Dieters are volume eaters, and many processed foods offer little bang for the buck.

But here's the thing. I can tell you to avoid processed foods whenever possible, but I'm also a realist. I know you're busy. I know there are going to be many days when you're going to look for the path of least resistance. Shopping for food and preparing meals takes time, and that may not always be an option for you. If you're short on time, keeping your weight in check can be challenging.

The real question isn't whether your food has been cooked, baked, fermented, canned, frozen, mashed, or ground, but whether the food delivers great taste and lots of nutrition and leaves you feeling satisfied without doing you harm. Below is a short list of some great-tasting, light processed and packaged foods. Keep in mind that many processed and packaged foods come in large, unmeasured portions. It can be difficult to know what a serving size is. So, whenever possible, purchase these foods in single-serving packages or get the smallest portion available.

1. Oikos Caramel Greek Yogurt
2. Plum Organics Mish Mash Fruit Purees
3. Tyson Grilled Ready Roasted Chicken Breast Pieces
4. Trader Joe's Pulled Chicken Breast
5. Starkist Yellow Fin Tuna in Water
6. DiGiornio 200-Calorie Portion Cheese Pizza
7. Emerald 100-Calorie Almond Packs
8. V8 Low-Sodium Vegetable Juice
9. Wasa Light Rye Crackers
10. Oscar Mayer Deli Fresh Cold Cuts

Never Skip a Meal Again

IN MANY CIRCLES, SKIPPING MEALS MAY SEEM LIKE AN ATTRACTIVE way to lose weight, but this is a classic example of the cure being worse than the disease. The consequences of skipping meals can include inadequate nutrition, altered metabolism, and constant dips and spikes in blood sugar. Blood sugar drops cause you to feel sluggish and tired and wreak havoc with insulin. To compensate, your body signals your brain to reach for whatever food will restore your blood sugar as quickly as possible. This puts you at risk of falling back on a bad boyfriend food, since these naughty men are almost always high in carbohydrates and simple sugars.

On the Skinny Jeans Diet, you have three meals and two to three snacks a day, which means you're eating something approximately every three hours.

Breakfast: Though it's called brea*kfast* and literally follows an 8- to 12-hour break from eating, don't feel the need to force-feed yourself by a certain time. I have a client who gets nauseous if she eats before 10:00 in the morning. Don't set an arbitrary deadline, but do try to eat something before noon, even if it's just a small meal.

Lunch: I advise clients to have lunch by 2:00 in the afternoon at the latest to avoid a blood sugar crash and to have the energy needed for the afternoon's activities. Ideally, lunch should include a combination of lean protein, complex carbohydrates, and fat. This simple combination of macronutrients will keep you satisfied and give you enough energy to get over any afternoon hurdle.

Dinner: As with lunch, I advise clients to eat dinner by a certain time, usually no later than 7:00 at night—not because I'm concerned about their metabolism or energy level, but so that they eat before they're physically hungry. It's no different than advising you to drink before you're thirsty. Eating before hunger strikes will keep cravings at bay and prevent you from overeating.

Boring Can Be Good

A MAJORITY OF MY CLIENTS FIND THAT CHOOSING FROM THEIR own personal list of great-tasting low-calorie foods helps limit temptation and keep them on the straight and narrow. A groundbreaking study by the National Weight Control Registry found that people who lose 30 pounds or more and keep the weight off for at least a year "limit their exposure to temptations and have a repertoire of healthy foods they pull from regularly." As I've mentioned several times, variety stimulates consumption, so limiting your choices is the best way to avoid being put in a compromising position.

The Skinny Jeans Diet General Rules to Remember

- **One fruit choice every day should be an apple.** The others can be whatever you prefer.
- **Take a daily multivitamin/mineral supplement.**
- **Drink lots of noncaffeinated, zero-calorie liquids.**

Caffeine is a diuretic, so caffeinated beverages don't hydrate you, and even low levels of dehydration can show up as hunger. It's fine to drink caffeinated beverages—but just keep this in mind.

- **Always keep a shopping list on hand so you are prepared.**
- **Plan meals and snacks.** You should know what you are having for dinner . . . at breakfast.
- **Never eat when you're hungry.** If you've waited until you're hungry, you have waited too long to eat. Your blood sugar has dipped and hunger-stimulating hormones have been activated. Eat every three to four hours.
- **Eat your meals and snacks about the same time every day.** Your body will soon know exactly when to expect its next meal, so you're more likely to have fewer cravings, do less emotional eating, and avoid off-the-cuff snacking.
- **Weigh and measure all foods.** Use measuring spoons or cups and a food scale to do this.
- **Use smaller dishes and smaller utensils.** Eating off a salad plate will make your portions look like more, and eating with smaller utensils will make you take smaller bites.
- **Eat in the right order.** Start with greens! Eat vegetables first to naturally have more of them and ultimately eat fewer calories at your meal.
- **Have an action plan to help you achieve small and specific goals.** Do you tend to nosh while prepping dinner? Then chew gum or snack on raw carrots or strips of pepper. Do you have carpool duty right at dinnertime? Get your meal prepared beforehand so it will be ready upon your return. Action always feels better than inaction!

- **No cruise control eating.** Much of our daily eating happens on cruise control—sticking a hand in the cereal box, grabbing a doughnut with coffee, licking the last of the batter from the bowl before rinsing it. These small habits can spell diet disaster. Picture all those bites, licks, and tastes going into a Ziploc bag, then add up the bag's calories at the end of the day. Pay attention!

Getting Started

AS YOU READ THROUGH THE MEAL PLANS, SHOPPING LISTS, AND DE-licious recipes that follow, I want you to stop and think for a moment about why you're reading this book. If you're like most of my clients, you're sick and tired of being sick and tired. You've had enough of having your life revolve around food. You're exhausted by the prospect of another day spent obsessing about the scale, how your clothes fit, and the way your face looks in the mirror. You're tired of playing musical chairs in your doctor's office and scouring the plus-size racks at the local department store only to end up in tears in the store's dressing room. You've reached the point where you simply can't count, measure, or weigh another calorie or gram of fat or carbohydrate.

The Skinny Jeans Diet offers freedom from the insanity and obsession that haunt the lives of most dieters. You'll finally be in control of your life with food. Nothing feels better than that—well, except maybe fitting into your favorite clothes!

The great Taoist philosopher Lao Tzu said, "To the mind that is still, the whole universe surrenders." Seldom can we control our circumstances, and even our efforts can be difficult to manage. But we can always control our reactions. If your bad boyfriend food is chocolate and your husband one night walks in the door with a deluxe box of Godiva truffles, you can scream, threaten divorce, or hurl the box across the room. Or you can calmly employ any of the creative strategies in this book and enjoy a much better outcome. Remember, there's no greater gift you can give yourself than knowing you have the power to remove the specter of unhappiness that food has caused in your life and replace it with a healthier, happier, and thinner you.

TO THY OWN SELF BE TRUE

Any diet will work . . . if you stay on it. The key is to make the diet your own. Make it fit with your food preferences, behaviors, and habits. Do what you need to do to stay on the plan without feeling deprived. If you don't like cereal in the morning because it activates carbohydrate cravings for you, choose a high-protein breakfast, such as eggs. If you like to have a small treat, such as a piece of fruit or a 100-calorie frozen novelty, before going to sleep, please do so.

The Skinny Jeans Diet is designed to give people more calories later in the day, as that seems to be our cultural preference. However, if you like to have more of your calories at lunch than at dinner, then feel free to switch around the lunch and dinner meals. Prefer eating an early dinner with the kids rather than a late one with your spouse? Then have dinner at 5:00 P.M. with the kids and your evening treat with your significant other later in the evening. Don't feel the need for a mid-morning snack because of your work and child care schedule? Then have the snack later in the day when you would enjoy it more.

Make the Skinny Jeans Diet your own. This personalization of the food plan is very important, since you'll have to come up with your own food plan and routine when it comes time for maintenance. The Skinny Jeans Diet won't leave you hanging, though. We give you guidelines to get you through.

~~~~

CHAPTER 9

Phase I: The Skinny Jeans Three-Day Detox Plan

THE SKINNY JEANS THREE-DAY DETOX PLAN IS A WAY TO GET going on your weight loss, stat! The detox diet is easy to follow and works great for people who are out of control with their food choices and need a strict, structured plan with limited variety. It's aggressive enough to give you a jump-start so you lose weight quickly and get motivated to keep going. Women may lose as much as three to five pounds on the Three-Day Detox (and one to two pounds per week thereafter in Phase II, the main diet phase). Men may lose more. (Men have more testosterone, which gives them a weight loss advantage.) Part of that loss will be water. Also, your age and metabolic rate will influence your rate of weight loss.

The caloric budget for the detox is approximately 1,000 calories. Follow the Skinny Jeans Detox for no more than three days.

If you've had it with strict diets, then the detox phase may not be for you. You may want to jump ahead and go right to the main Master

Weight Loss Plan. For the rest of you, here are some rules to remember for the Skinny Jeans Three-Day Detox Plan:

- If at any time you feel discomfort or deprived on the detox diet, move to Phase II, the Master Weight Loss Plan.
- There are no starchy carbohydrates on the detox diet. Those foods are introduced in Phase II (the Master Weight Loss Plan).
- You can eat food throughout the day on the detox diet, except for following the fruit-only guideline between breakfast and lunch. For example, if you prefer to switch up your lunch and dinner meals, that's okay.
- Follow the Skinny Jeans Diet detox for no more than three days.
- On the detox, your choices are a limited selection of foods from the different food groups. Within any one food group, you can substitute foods for each other, in the portion sizes shown for each.

Refer to the food lists starting on page 232 for details on particular foods.

Breakfast (Anytime Before Noon)

- 2 to 3 fruit servings (no bananas, grapes, pineapple, mango, or cherries)

Lunch (Anytime Before 2:00 P.M.)

- 4 ounces lean protein (tofu, chicken, turkey, seafood, shellfish); or 3 ounces reduced-fat cheese; or ½ cup beans/legumes; or 2 eggs (3 egg whites + ¼ cup liquid egg substitute = 1 egg)
- Unlimited salad and/or nonstarchy cooked vegetable
- 1 teaspoon oil; or 2 tablespoons low-fat dressing (any dressing with 50 calories or less per serving); or 10 olives; or 1 serving of another fat from the fat food list

Midafternoon Snack (Choose One Snack per Day)

- Questbar Protein Bar
- 1 serving of fruit with a 100-calorie nut pack
- 1 apple with 2 teaspoons any peanut or nut butter; or 1 tablespoon Better'n Peanut Butter; or 2 tablespoons powdered peanut butter (such as PB2); or 1 light string cheese
- 1 nonfat (Greek is preferable) yogurt (100 to 140 calories) with either a fruit serving or a 100-calorie pack of almonds or 1 light string cheese
- 2 tablespoons hummus with carrots or other vegetable
- Gnu FiberLove Bar with a fruit serving
- Any nutrition bar that has 160 to 210 calories or less and at least 10 grams of protein and 5 grams of fiber per bar (favorites include Questbar Protein Bars, Kashi Go Lean Protein and Fiber Bars, KIND Bars, Special K Protein Bars)

Dinner

- 5 ounces lean protein or 1 cup beans/legumes
- Unlimited nonstarchy vegetables
- 1 teaspoon fat (butter or oil) or other fat serving from the fat food list

Evening Snack

- 1 grapefruit (if you cannot or prefer not to eat grapefruit, an orange, peach, plum, nectarine, or 2 tangerines may be substituted)

ADJUSTMENTS FOR MEN IN PHASE I: THE SKINNY JEANS THREE-DAY DETOX PLAN

- At lunch, have 6 ounces of protein (2 extra ounces).
- At dinner, have 8 ounces of protein (3 extra ounces).

~~~~~~~~

CHAPTER 10

Phase II: The Skinny Jeans Diet Master Weight Loss Plan

A T THE END OF THE THREE-DAY DETOX PHASE, PHASE II
kicks in. The Master Weight Loss Plan will take you straight
to your chosen weight!

Breakfast

Choose one of the options below:

1. *PB&J sandwich*
   - 100-calorie sandwich thin; or 100-calorie high-fiber wrap; or 100-calorie whole grain English muffin
   - 2 teaspoons peanut or nut butter; or 1 tablespoon Better'n Peanut Butter; or 2 tablespoons powdered peanut butter (such as PB2)
   - 1 teaspoon low-sugar jam

2. *Grilled cheese sandwich*
   - 100-calorie sandwich thin; or 100-calorie high-fiber wrap; or 100-calorie whole grain English muffin
   - 1 ounce light string cheese, peeled and melted
3. *1 egg* (3 egg whites + ¼ cup liquid egg substitute= 1 egg), cooked (with 100-calorie high-fiber wrap)
4. *2 eggs* (3 egg whites + ¼ cup liquid egg substitute = 1 egg)
5. 100- to 140-calorie nonfat yogurt (Greek is preferable) with one fruit serving
6. *Cold cereal and milk*
   - 1 cup high-fiber cereal (120 calories or less per 1 cup serving; favorites include Special K Protein Plus, Fiber One, Kashi Heart to Heart Honey Toasted Cereal, or multiple varieties of Cheerios)
   - ¼ cup skim milk or unsweetened almond milk
   - 1 fruit serving
7. *1 cup cooked cereal* (no sugar added) . . .
   - . . . made with water or unsweetened almond milk
   - 1 fruit serving
8. *Any breakfast that is 180 calories or less*

Midmorning Snack

- One fruit serving

Choose one from each of the following categories (note that to lose more weight, you have the option to forgo a complex carbohydrate):

- *Protein:* 4 ounces lean protein; or ½ cup beans/legumes; or 1 vegetable burger; or 3 ounces reduced-fat cheese; or 2 eggs (3 egg whites + ¼ cup liquid egg substitute = 1 egg)
- *Vegetable:* Unlimited nonstarchy cooked or raw vegetables (see page 235)
- *Fat:* 1 teaspoon fat, such as oil, butter, or mayonnaise; or 2 tablespoons low-calorie dressing (approximately 50 calories or less per serving); or 1 fat serving from the fat food list (page 240)
- *100-calorie complex carbohydrate (optional):* 3 to 5 flatbreads (i.e.: Ak-Mak, Wasa, Kavli, Trader Joe's, GG Scandinavian Crisp breads); or a 100-calorie sandwich thin; or a 100-calorie high fiber wrap; or 2 slices low-calorie bread; or 15 oriental rice crackers (i.e.; Asian Gourmet); or 1 complex carbohydrate serving from the Complex Carbohydrate food list (page 238)

Midafternoon Snack

Choose a single serving of fruit (preferably an apple), and then any one of the following:

- 2 teaspoons peanut or nut butter
- 1 tablespoon Better'n Peanut Butter or 2 tablespoons powdered peanut butter
- 100-calorie individual pack of nuts
- 2 tablespoons hummus with a nonstarchy vegetable
- 6 to 8 ounces 0 percent nonfat yogurt (100 to 140 calories per container)
- 4 ounces nonfat frozen yogurt
- 1 light cheese stick
- 100-calorie bag of 94 percent fat-free popcorn
- Soy or popped chips (100 to 150 calories per single-serving bag), such as Glenny's, Pop Chips, Quaker Rice Crisps, or Way Smarter Chips
- 1 Clif KidZ Bar (130 calories) or Gnu FiberLove Bar (140 calories)
- 1 Alba 70 Snack Shake

Note that you may also choose to have a 160- to 210-calorie nutrition bar as your afternoon snack. If you choose this option, you will have to forgo having any fruit with it. The bar must have 160 to 210 calories and at least 10 grams of protein and 5 grams of fiber. Favorites include:

- Questbar protein bars
- KIND bars
- Kashi Protein and Fiber bars
- Special K protein bars

Dinner

Choose one of these two meal options:

1. *Protein, Vegetable, and Fat Meal:*
   - 5 ounces lean protein; or 1 cup beans/legumes; or 2 vegetable burgers (120 calories or less per patty); or 4 ounces reduced-fat cheese
   - Unlimited nonstarchy cooked or raw vegetables
   - 1 teaspoon oil or butter; or 2 tablespoons light butter (in other words, 1 fat serving from the fat food list)
2. *Frozen dinner meal:*
   - 300-calorie-or-less frozen dinner meal—for example, Weight Watchers, Kashi, Whole Foods 365, Lean Cuisine, Lightlife, or Amy's Organic
   - Large amount of nonstarchy vegetables mixed in

Evening Snack

Choose half a grapefruit or a whole grapefruit nightly—plus an Optional Free 100! Please note that if you cannot eat grapefruit, or prefer not to, an orange, peach, plum, or 2 tangerines can be substituted.

The Daily Optional Free 100! is a 100-calorie free snack each day, such as a 100-calorie frozen novelty, a 100-calorie protein bar, or a 100-calorie snack bag. Please note that you can "bank" these calories and use the cumulative calories at one meal or over the course of one day. However, your Free 100! choice should never be a bad boyfriend food, even if it comes in a 100-calorie portion. That's a snack that could activate cravings for your bad boy, and you'll find the frequency of this choice—and ultimately quantity—increasing. Stick to a nice guy alternative!

ADJUSTMENTS FOR MEN IN PHASE II:
THE SKINNY JEANS MASTER WEIGHT LOSS PLAN

- At lunch, have 6 ounces of protein.
- At dinner, have 8 ounces of protein plus 1 small baked or sweet potato; or ½ cup of starchy vegetables or whole grains; or 1 other complex carbohydrate serving from the food list.

A few pointers:

- To accelerate weight loss, you can omit the optional complex carbohydrate with lunch and/or the daily Optional Free 100! Both are included in these sample meal plans.
- You can alternate any meal and snack to best suit your food preferences and routine.
- The Skinny Jeans Diet Recipes start on page 246. Any Skinny Jeans Diet Recipe can be used on the meal plan. A lunch should be approximately 230 to 250 calories and dinner should be approximately 300 calories. As long as you

stick to the serving sizes and make sure they do not exceed those calorie approximations, you'll be fine. For example, if you want to eat Speedy, Skinny Potato Fries (page 273), pair them with the Easiest Roasted Veggies, Ever! (page 268) to come up with a 300-calorie meal (see sample day 7, page 220).

- If you cannot or choose to not eat an evening grapefruit, you may eat a peach, plum, or nectarine as an alternative. Just keep in mind that grapefruit is a diuretic and takes the water weight off!

Day 1

BREAKFAST
Peanut Butter and Jelly Sandwich

2 tablespoons Better'n Peanut Butter or 2 tablespoons
   powdered peanut butter
1 teaspoon Smucker's Sugar-Free Jam
1 Arnold Select 100-Calorie Sandwich Thin

MIDMORNING SNACK
1 peach

LUNCH
Chicken Caesar Salad

3 ounces roasted chicken breast
2 tablespoons shredded Parmesan cheese
Large romaine lettuce, shredded
2 tablespoons Marie's Yogurt Dressing, Caesar Parmesan
3 Ak-Mak Whole Wheat Crackers

MIDAFTERNOON SNACK

1 nonfat Greek yogurt

1 apple

DINNER

Salmon and Mashed Potatoes

5 ounces Simple Salmon (page 254)

1 serving Mock Mashed Potatoes (page 269)

1 teaspoon light margarine (such as Brummel and Brown Buttery Spread)

EVENING SNACK

1 100-calorie Trader Joe's Milk Chocolate Bar

½ to 1 grapefruit

Day 2

BREAKFAST
Grilled Cheese

1 light string cheese, peeled
1 La Tortilla Factory High-Fiber 100-Calorie Wrap

MIDMORNING SNACK

1 cup blueberries

LUNCH
Roast Beef Sandwich

4 ounces lean roast beef
2 slices light bread
1 teaspoon ketchup (free)
Lettuce and tomato slices
1 cup raw baby carrots
1 cup red bell pepper slices
2 tablespoons salsa, for dipping (free)

MIDAFTERNOON SNACK

1 bag 94 percent fat-free microwave popcorn (100 calories)
1 apple

DINNER

1 serving Quick, Skinny Chili (page 255)
2 cups kale chips (Roast kale with nonstick spray, kosher salt, and 1 teaspoon olive oil at 425 degrees for 5–7 minutes; flip halfway through cooking.)

EVENING SNACK

1 Healthy Choice Fudge Bar
½ to 1 grapefruit

Day 3

BREAKFAST

1 Mug Egg Scramble (page 250)

MIDMORNING SNACK

1 nectarine

LUNCH

Tuna Salad Sandwich

4 ounces water-packed tuna

1 tablespoon light mayonnaise

1 tablespoon Hellmann's Dijonnaise Mustard-Mayonnaise Blend

1 Joseph's Flax, Oat Bran and Whole Wheat Lavash Bread (100 calories for entire lavash)

1 cup chopped celery and onion, or to taste

1 cup cucumber dipped in Dijon-style mustard

MIDAFTERNOON SNACK

1 Clif KidZ Chocolate Chip Bar
1 apple

DINNER

1 Steak Stir-Fry (page 256)

EVENING SNACK

1 Jell-O Mousse Temptations Chocolate Mousse
½ to 1 grapefruit

Day 4

BREAKFAST

1 non-fat or low-fat Greek yogurt (100–140 calories)
1 cup blueberries and raspberries, mixed

MIDMORNING SNACK

½ banana

LUNCH

Turkey Sandwich

3 ounces sliced turkey breast
1 ounce sliced reduced-fat Swiss cheese
2 tablespoons low-fat Russian dressing (50 calories or less per 2
  tablespoons)
1 La Tortilla Factory Smart & Delicious 100-Calorie Tortilla
½ sliced tomato
1 cup jicama dipped in honey mustard to taste

MIDAFTERNOON SNACK

1 100-calorie pack of Emerald Cocoa Roast Almonds
1 Skinny Baked Apple (page 274)

DINNER

1 serving Cauliflower "Flatbread" (page 257)
2 cups eggplant sautéed in ½ cup light tomato sauce (60 calories or less per ½ cup)

EVENING SNACK

Skinny S'more (page 275)
½ to 1 grapefruit

Day 5

BREAKFAST

1 Berry Good Smoothie (page 249)

MIDMORNING SNACK

1 pear

LUNCH

Hot Dogs

2 reduced-fat hot dogs

1 low-calorie hot dog roll (use only 1 hot dog roll and eat the other hot dog solo)

Mustard

1 cup sauerkraut

1 cup shredded cabbage mixed with 2 tablespoons reduced-calorie ranch dressing (50 calories or less per 2-tablespoon serving)

MIDAFTERNOON SNACK

1 Clif KidZ Bar, any flavor

1 apple

DINNER

1 serving Lemon Chicken Thighs with Olives and Capers
(page 262)

1 serving Easiest Spaghetti Squash Ever! (page 260)

EVENING SNACK

1 Weight Watchers Snack-Size Vanilla/Chocolate Ice Cream
Sandwich

½ to 1 grapefruit

Day 6

BREAKFAST

1 Skinny Jeans Diet Alba 70 Shake (page 248)

MIDMORNING SNACK

1 orange

LUNCH

1 serving Skinny Egg White Salad (page 252)

MIDAFTERNOON SNACK

1 Gnu FiberLove Bar, any flavor
½ cup no-sugar-added applesauce

DINNER

1 serving Skinny Meatloaf (page 258)
1 serving Skinny Glazed Carrots (page 272)

EVENING SNACK

1 Skinny Baked Pear (page 276)
1 Jell-0 sugar-free gelatin dessert (free)
½ to 1 grapefruit

Day 7

BREAKFAST

1 cup cooked oatmeal made with ½ cup unsweetened almond
   milk or water
1 tablespoon raisins

MIDMORNING SNACK

2 tangerines

LUNCH

1 BBQ Chicken Pizza (page 251)
1 cup steamed spinach with kosher salt

MIDAFTERNOON SNACK

1 Morning Peanut Butter Cup Sandwich (page 247)
1 apple

DINNER

1 to 3 servings Easiest Roasted Vegetables Ever! (page 268)
1 serving Speedy, Skinny Potato Fries (page 273)
2 tablespoons ketchup

EVENING SNACK

100-calorie pack of Sarri's Chocolate Pretzels Slims
½ to 1 grapefruit

〜〜〜

CHAPTER 11

Phase III: The Skinny Jeans Diet Maintenance Plan

CONGRATULATIONS! YOU'VE REACHED YOUR WEIGHT GOAL and changed your thinking to change your eating. The Skinny Jeans Three-Day Detox gave you an encouraging and aggressive jump-start, the Master Weight Loss Plan guided you to finally fitting into your pants, and now it's time to stay thin—forever.

There are more than just the two states of eating: either on a diet or not. The first essential step in weight maintenance is eliminating the artificial boundary between weight loss and weight maintenance. You'll use the same strategies and effort to maintain your weight that you used to lose it. For most people, the difference between the two is only a couple of hundred calories. That's a baked potato added to dinner, half a sandwich with your lunch salad, or a few more bites of dessert. Here are some tips to help you survive the transition from weight loss to weight maintenance and finally become one of the It Girls.

1. Weigh yourself every day or every other day.
2. If you start to gain weight, you must reverse these gains immediately. Increase your intake of white-colored fish and green, leafy vegetables. Cut back on starchy carbohydrates.
3. Get active in your daily life. This will increase your metabolic rate, relieve stress, and improve your overall well-being. When you feel happier, you won't use food as much to fight the blues.
4. Remember that fitting into your skinny jeans has little to do with what you're eating and everything to do with how you're thinking. Don't reconnect with your bad boyfriend foods, do manage your food environment, and do form a game plan for high-risk situations.

Suggested Maintenance Plans

- *Women:* Add 100 to 200 calories per day. I recommend doing this by adding one complex carbohydrate serving and one fat serving to your evening meal.
- *Men:* Add 200 to 300 calories per day. I recommend doing this by adding one complex carbohydrate serving to your lunch meal and two complex carbohydrate servings and one fat serving to your dinner meal.

Examples of a Complex Carbohydrate Serving

- 1 medium baked or sweet potato
- ½ cup pasta, rice, or other cooked grains
- 1 medium whole-grain dinner roll or 1 ear of corn
- 1 hamburger or hot dog bun
- 1 100-calorie flatbread, sandwich thin, or English muffin

Examples of a Fat Serving

- 2 tablespoons light salad dressing or marinade
- 1 tablespoon butter or oil
- 2 tablespoons butter spread, such as Brummel and Brown

Cheap Cheat

YOU HAVE AN EXTRA 100 TO 200 CALORIES PER DAY. ENJOY them how you wish, but make sure you know the calories you're consuming—and you still have to keep away from bad boyfriend foods!

CHAPTER 12

Consider the Alternatives: The Skinny Jeans Diet Top 75 BFFs

N O ONE WANTS TO MISS OUT ON A PARTY. DIETERS ARE NO different. Indeed, few things cause dieters to throw in the towel faster than the sense that they're missing out on the fun and pleasure of eating. Imagine someone telling you that you can never have another cookie, piece of chocolate, or potato chip. Hello? You might as well ban me from wearing high heels and lipstick.

Fortunately, in today's vast food universe there's an alternative for every naughty, high-calorie bad boy food you love. Below is a list of the Skinny Jeans Diet BFFs, or Best Friend Foods. These foods have helped my clients fend off the sense that they're being handed a life sentence. They'll give you satisfaction and pleasure without a lot of excess guilt and excess calories.

Whatever food you choose, just be certain that it's not an alternative that could reactivate cravings and trigger overeating. For example,

I have a client who abuses chocolate, no matter what form it takes. Even an innocent little mug of watered-down diet hot chocolate will send her over the edge. Long ago, she made the decision that it was better not to have chocolate in her life. It's not that she can't have chocolate. Rather, it just didn't work for her.

Here are my top 75 Skinny Jeans Diet BFFs—like real-life friends, they'll get you through plenty of sticky situations! Most of these are available quite widely in grocery stores and online, but I've included sourcing information on a few that might be more obscure.

Beverages

1. Alba 70 Snack Shake Mix
2. Almond Breeze Unsweetened Almond Milk

Sauces, Spreads, and Dressings

1. Better'n Peanut Butter
2. Maple Grove Farms of Vermont Fat-Free Salad Dressings
3. Mr. Yoshida's Marinade and Cooking Sauce (Costco or Sam's Club)
4. Pam Olive Oil Non-Stick Spray
5. Smucker's Sugar-Free Jam
6. Kraft Single-Packet Fat-Free Salad Dressings (minimus.biz)

7. Justin's 80-Calorie Honey Peanut Butter packets (justinsnutbutter.com)
8. Trader Joe's Fat-Free Sesame Soy Ginger Vinaigrette
9. KC Masterpiece Steakhouse Marinade
10. DennyMike's BBQ Rubs and Enhancers (dennymikes. com or Whole Foods)
11. Trader Joe's Organic Marinara Sauce
12. Frank's Red Hot Sauce
13. Marie's All-Natural Yogurt Parmesan Caesar Dressing
14. Log Cabin Sugar Pancake Syrup
15. Best Life Buttery Spread
16. Hellmann's/Best Foods Dijonnaise
17. Tribe Hummus, individual serving cups
18. Good Neighbor Simply Zero Organic Hummus (Whole Foods)
19. PB2 powdered peanut butter

Crackers, Chips, and Other Snacks

1. Orville Redenbacher's Smartpop! Popcorn, 100-calorie mini-bags
2. Emerald 100-calorie nut packs
3. Asian Gourmet Rice Crackers
4. Kavli Crispy Thin All-Natural Whole-Grain Crispbread
5. Glenny's Soy Crisps
6. Popchips 100-calorie snack packs

7. Sarri's 100-Calorie Pretzel Slim (sarriscandies.com)
8. Cape Cod 40 Percent Reduced-Fat 100-Calorie Potato Chip packs
9. Sea Snax Seaweed Snacks

Cereals and Bars

1. Cheerios—Multigrain, Cinnamon, Dulce de Leche, Peanut Butter, and Chocolate Flavor
2. Special K Protein Plus Cereal
3. Quaker Puffed Wheat Cereal
4. Kashi Heart to Heart Honey Toasted Cereal
5. Chocolite Bars (healthsmartfoods.com)
6. Questbar Protein Bar
7. Yasso Frozen Greek Yogurt Bars

Pasta and Bread

1. Fiber Gourmet Pasta (www.fibergourmet.com)
2. La Tortilla Factory Smart & Delicious Low-Carb, High-Fiber, 100-Calorie Wraps
3. Kim's Light Bagels
4. Flatout Foldit Flatbreads
5. Nasoya Pasta Zero Plus Shiratake Tofu Noodles
6. Joseph's Flax, Oat Bran, and Whole Wheat Lavash

Fruits and Vegetables

1. Pink Lady Apples
2. Green Giant Cut Leaf Spinach and Low-Fat Butter Sauce
3. Birds Eye Steamfresh Vegetables

Dairy

1. Chobani 0 Percent Greek Yogurt
2. Laughing Cow Light Cheese Wedges
3. Weight Watchers Light String Cheese
4. Egg Beaters Liquid Egg Substitute
5. Athenos Reduced-Fat Crumbled Feta Cheese
6. Laughing Cow Mini Babybel Cheese Round

Main Meals

1. Garden Lites Souffles
2. Dr. Praeger's California Veggie Burgers
3. Trader Joe's Italian-Style Chicken Sausage
4. Tyson Grilled Ready Roasted Chicken Breast, chopped or strips
5. Oscar Mayer Deli Fresh Shaved Turkey Breast, Chicken Breast, Ham, and Roast Beef, slices
6. Vitalicious Cheese and Tomato Vitapizza

7. Trader Joe's Pulled Chicken Breast

8. Laura's Lean Beef

9. Morning Star Farms Hickory BBQ Riblets

10. Dunkin Donuts Egg White Omelet Flatout, without cheese

11. Hebrew National 97 Percent Fat-Free Beef Franks

12. DiGiornio 200-Calorie-Portion Cheese Pizza

13. Trader Joe's Meatless Meatballs

14. Perdue Simple Smart Lightly Breaded Chicken

15. Amy's Brown Rice, Black-eyed Peas, and Veggies Bowl

Sweets

1. Trader Joe's 100-Calorie Milk or Dark Chocolate Bars

2. Fiber One 90-Calorie Brownies

3. Weight Watchers Snack-Size Frozen Novelties

4. Healthy Choice Fudge Bars

5. Funky Monkey Freeze-Dried Fruit

6. Splenda Sugar Blend

7. Q.bel Dark Chocolate Wafer Rolls

8. Skinny Cow Heavenly Crisp 110-Calorie Bars

Skinny Jeans Diet Top 10 Best Friend Bars

MANY OF MY DIETERS LIKE NUTRITION BARS AS AN AFTERNOON snack because they're convenient, they take away the need to think about food during the afternoon hours, and the calorie counting has already been done for them. Look for bars with 210 calories or less, about 5 grams of fiber, and at least 10 grams of protein. The combo of fiber and protein is super-filling, and the calories will help keep you in your skinny jeans.

Some of the following bars have less protein but much more fiber, so they still make the list:

1. Gnu FiberLove Bars
2. Questbar Protein Bars
3. Kashi Go Lean Protein and Fiber Bars
4. Kashi Go Lean Crunchy! Bars
5. Clif KidZBars
6. KIND Bars
7. Perfectly Simple by Zone Perfect
8. Larabars
9. Nature Valley Protein Chewy Bars
10. Special K Protein Meal Bars

CHAPTER 13

The Skinny Jeans Diet Food Lists

List 1: Lean Protein Foods

THE FOLLOWING FOODS ALL EQUAL 1 OUNCE OF PROTEIN:

- 1 ounce skinless, boneless chicken or turkey meat (white or dark meat is okay)
- 1 ounce fish or shellfish, any type, fresh or frozen, unbreaded
- 1 ounce tuna, water-packed
- 1 ounce lean meat (beef eye of round, top round or tip round, flank steak, sirloin steak, veal chops/veal roast, beef tenderloin, skirt steak, pork tenderloin, boneless sirloin chop, or boneless loin roast)
- 1 ounce extra-lean ground beef or turkey
- 1 ounce low-fat luncheon meat (no more than 50 calories per ounce)
- 1 ounce lean ham
- 1 ounce Canadian or turkey bacon

- 1 ounce reduced-fat hot dogs (no more than 50 calories per ounce)
- 2 medium sardines, canned with no oil
- 1 large egg
- 3 egg whites
- ¼ cup egg substitute
- ¼ cup 1 percent or nonfat cottage cheese or ricotta cheese
- 1 Laughing Cow Mini Babybel Cheese Round
- 1 wedge Laughing Cow Light Cheese
- 1 light string cheese (for example, Polly-O Lite, Weight Watchers)
- 1 ounce reduced-fat or fat-free cheese (Fat-free cheese contains approximately 50 calories per ounce; reduced-fat cheese contains about 50 to 70 calories per ounce, more than other protein sources. Thus, 3 ounces of reduced-fat cheese = 4 ounces of protein.)
- 1 tablespoon grated Parmesan cheese
- 1 tablespoon crumbled feta or goat cheese
- ¼ cup nonfat yogurt
- ¼ cup skim milk; or unsweetened almond milk; or light soymilk
- 1 teaspoon peanut or nut butter
- 1 tablespoon Better'n Peanut Butter (available at betternpeanutbutter.com or large retailers)
- 2 teaspoons hummus
- 1 vegetable burger (120 calories or less = 4 ounces of protein)
- ¼ cup cooked beans/legumes (chickpeas, kidney beans, white beans, split or black-eyed peas, lentils)

Important note about beans: Half a cup of cooked beans contains about 80 to 100 calories, which is more than other protein sources. Unlike most of the other protein foods, however, beans contain only a trace of fat, making them an excellent substitute for meat or cheese. Most people will find a serving of between half a cup and a cup of beans—the protein equivalent of three to five ounces of meat—very filling. If you're using beans as your protein choice, have half a cup at lunch and/or one cup at dinner to keep calories under control.

A few pointers to keep in mind:

1. All meats, poultry, and fish should be weighed when they are cooked. You'll lose approximately one ounce of weight after cooking. So, to make life more convenient, ask the butcher or fish store to portion out one ounce more, knowing the meat or fish will lose weight in cooking. For example, ask for a six-ounce portion of raw salmon, knowing it will yield five ounces for dinner after being cooked.

2. Foods should be cooked without added fat. Use an oil sprayer or nonstick cooking spray to moisten food. Never pour oil or fat over food.

3. It's okay to marinate your food. No one is fat because they marinated their chicken. Just be smart and don't pour extra marinade onto your portion or dip your food into a lot of marinade or condiments (like ketchup).

List 2: Vegetables

REMEMBER THAT VEGETABLES SHOULD TAKE UP THE MOST REAL estate on your plate. And also don't forget that, when you pick veggies from this first list, portion sizes are unlimited!

- Lettuce, any type, shredded
- Cabbage, any type
- Celery
- Cucumber
- Mushroom
- Pepper (green, red, yellow), medium-size
- Radish
- Spinach
- Bean sprouts
- Zucchini
- Eggplant
- Asparagus
- Artichoke
- Beans (green, yellow, Italian)
- Broccoli
- Brussels sprouts
- Cauliflower
- Okra
- Pea pods
- Summer squash
- Spaghetti squash
- Tomato

Eat the vegetables in the following list in moderation, i.e., one or two servings per day (one serving = 1 cup raw or ½ cup cooked):

- Tomato/spaghetti sauce (50 calories or less per ½ cup)
- Tomato juice or vegetable juice cocktail (½ cup)
- Onion
- Carrot
- Jicama
- Kohlrabi
- Parsnip
- Rutabaga
- Turnip
- Water chestnuts

A few pointers:

1. Vegetables may be fresh, frozen, or canned (but be cautious of canned veggies, which are higher in sodium).
2. Do not use added fats or sauces other than those recommended.
3. Eat your water! Veggies are high in water content, and water has zero calories. (But you knew that!) That is why they must take up the most real estate on your plate. You can have plenty of food, feel full, and cut calories substantially. More veggies + feeling full = easier weight loss and a happier dieter!

List 3: Fruits

IMPORTANT NOTE ABOUT FRUIT CHOICES: ONE FRUIT CHOICE every day should be an apple. Many dieters find that having the apple in the afternoon with their snack selection helps ward off afternoon grazing. The other fruit choices are up to you. One serving of raw fruit is equal to:

- 1 medium apple
- 1 orange
- 1 pear
- 1 peach or nectarine
- 1 kiwi
- ½ banana
- ½ grapefruit
- 1 cup cubed cantaloupe or honeydew
- 15 small grapes
- 12 cherries
- 1 cup cubed pineapple (or ⅓ cup canned in its own juices)
- 1 cup strawberries, blueberries, raspberries, or blackberries
- ½ cup fruit juice
- ½ cup unsweetened applesauce
- 1 cup cubed mango
- 1 cup cubed papaya
- 2 plums
- 2 tangerines
- 1 cup cubed watermelon

One serving of dried fruit is equal to:

- 4 apple rings
- 4 dried apricots
- 3 medium prunes
- 1 tablespoon raisins
- 3 medium dates

Important note about fruit: Remember that variety stimulates consumption? When it comes to eating fruit, however, variety can be a good thing. When you bring home several different colors and varieties of fruit, you may be more likely to eat it. Why? We are psychologically primed to want variety. Studies show that people ate 47 percent more of what was on their plate when the plate was filled with different-colored foods. Thus, a fruit salad is more appetizing than a single piece of melon!

List 4: Complex Carbohydrates

ONE SERVING OF EACH OF THE FOLLOWING FOODS HAS 80–120 CALories.

- 1 slice (1 ounce) regular, whole-grain bread
- 2 slices reduced-fat or light bread (approximately 45 calories per slice)
- 1 Kim's Light Bagel or Bagel Thin (approximately 110 calories)
- 1 high-fiber, 100-calorie wrap (8 grams of fiber or more per 100-calorie wrap), such as La Tortilla Factory Low-Carb

100-Calorie Wrap, Flatout Flatbreads, or Joseph's Oat Bran, Flax, and Wheat Lavash

- 1 100-calorie sandwich thin
- 1 low-calorie hamburger or hot dog bun (no more than 100 calories)
- 1 cup high-fiber cereal such as whole-grain O's (Cheerios) or bran flakes cereal (Special K Protein Plus, Fiber One) (approximately 120 calories per cup)
- ½ to 1 cup puffed cereal (unsweetened)
- 1 cup cooked cereal (unsweetened)
- ½ cup shredded wheat
- 1 board matzo (120 calories or less per board)
- 2 rice cakes
- 1 high-fiber pita (100 calories per pita)
- 1 high-fiber, 100-calorie light English muffin
- 1 frozen fat-free or light waffle (70 calories or less)
- 1 6-inch tortilla (100 calories per tortilla)
- 15 oriental rice crackers
- 3 to 5 flatbreads, such as Wasa, Finn Crisp, or Ak-Mak
- 5 slices Melba toast

A few pointers:

1. The higher the fiber in a complex carbohydrate, the fuller you will feel.
2. If a certain complex carbohydrate is a bad boyfriend for you, don't choose it!

For Phase III, Skinny Jeans Maintenance, you may add these starchy complex carbohydrates. You have the option to eat five ounces of protein with any of these selections for the dinner meal (e.g., five ounces of chicken with half a cup of rice), or three ounces of protein with two servings of any of these selections for the dinner meal (e.g., three ounces of flank steak with one medium baked potato).

- ½ cup corn or 1 small ear of corn (6 inches)
- ½ cup peas
- ½ cup winter squash (e.g., butternut)
- ½ medium sweet potato or baked potato (or 1 small)
- ½ cup brown rice, quinoa, couscous, or other high-fiber grain
- ½ cup high-fiber, whole-wheat pasta
- ½ cup starch-resistant pasta, such as Fiber Gourmet (www.fibergourmet.com)

List 5: Fats and Sugar

WITH FATS AND SUGAR, ONE SERVING HAS ABOUT 45 TO 50 CALOries, which is the equivalent of:

- 1 teaspoon regular margarine
- 1 tablespoon diet margarine (50 calories or less per tablespoon, as in Best Life Buttery Spread, Brummel and Brown Buttery Spread, and I Can't Believe It's Not Butter Light)
- 1 teaspoon regular mayonnaise
- 1 tablespoon reduced-fat mayonnaise

- 5 tablespoons nonfat mayonnaise (up to 2 tablespoons are free)
- 2 tablespoons reduced-calorie or light salad dressings (50 calories or less per 2-tablespoon serving)
- 1 teaspoon vegetable or olive oil
- ⅛ medium avocado
- 10 small or 5 large olives
- 50 calories (or less) of low-fat or nonfat sour cream
- 50 calories (or less) of cream cheese–style product (such as Neufchatel or fat-free cream cheese)
- 2 tablespoons reduced-calorie maple-flavored syrup
- 4 tablespoons sugar-free maple-flavored syrup
- 1 tablespoon jelly, jam, or preserves
- 1 tablespoon agave nectar
- 1 tablespoon honey

List 6: Free Foods

- Water
- Zero-calorie drinks and drink mixes
- Coffee or tea
- Bouillon, broth, or flavoring packets
- Sugar substitutes (e.g., Sweet-n-Low, Equal, Splenda, Truvia, Stevia)
- Low-calorie butter sprinkles or flakes (such as Butter Buds)
- Lemon or lime juice
- Hot sauce
- Flavor extracts (vanilla, lemon, and so on)

- Herbs and spices
- Horseradish
- Marinades (to marinate vegetables or protein foods)
- Up to ½ cup salsa
- 2 tablespoons ketchup or barbecue sauce
- 2 tablespoons relish
- Soy or Worcestershire sauce
- Mustard
- Vinegar
- Garlic
- Pickles
- Nonstick cooking spray (just be careful to spray, not coat)
- Sugar-free gelatin (2 individual cups or 1 envelope per day)
- Sugar-free gum or mints (up to 4 pieces per day)

List 7: Snack Foods

- Questbar Protein Bars (www.questnutrition.com)
- 1 bag 94 percent fat-free, 100-calorie popcorn or 5 cups air-popped popcorn
- 1 140-calorie (or less) high-fiber cereal snack or brownie bar (e.g., Fiber One or Fiber Plus)
- 1 Gnu FiberLove Bar
- 1 Clif KidZBar
- 1 100-calorie bag baked or popped chips (such as Popchips, Way Better Snack Chips, or Cape Cod 40 Percent Reduced-Fat 100-Calorie Potato Chip packs)
- 1 bag Soy Crisps (such as Glenny's)

- 1 Chocolite Protein Bar (www.healthsmartfoods.com)
- 2 teaspoons peanut or nut butter; or 1 tablespoon Better'n Peanut Butter; or 2 tablespoons powdered peanut butter (such as PB2)
- 1 100-calorie nut pack (e.g., Emerald or Blue Diamond)
- 2 tablespoons hummus with vegetables for dipping (or try Tribe individual hummus cups)
- 1 part-skim string cheese (70 calories or less)
- 6 to 8 ounces 0 percent nonfat yogurt (140 calories or less)
- 1 Alba 70 Snack Shake Mix

A few pointers:

1. Some people prefer to forgo their fruit in the afternoon and put the fruit calories toward eating a larger protein/fiber bar. If this is your preference, then you may choose a bar with a bigger size, weight, and calorie count. Look for bars that have 210 calories or less and at least 5 grams of fiber and 10 grams of protein. You will eat this bar as your one and only midafternoon snack (omitting the fruit).

2. Snacks versus treats—know the difference! Snacks offer nutrition and are meant to keep you full and get you from one meal to the next. They don't trigger cravings. Treats, on the other hand, are nutritionally void. Snacks are a regular and important part of your diet, and treats are eaten seldom and only on special occasions. When you start interchanging the two, you will get into trouble; i.e., greek yogurt, string cheese, peanut butter on an apple =

snacks. Frozen yogurt, pudding cups, baked chips, many 100 calorie packs = treats. Today, stop loading up on sweet treats and counting them as snacks. Get back to food basics.

3. For more mini–meal bar suggestions, see the Skinny Jeans Diet Top 10 Best Friend Bars, page 231.

List 8: Free 100! Food List

EVERY DAY ON THE SKINNY JEANS QUICK AND EASY DIET PLAN, you have 100 calories to spend however you please, provided it is not on a bad boyfriend food. These optional calories are known as your Free 100! and are put on the plan to prevent you from feeling deprived, which is the downfall of 95 percent of dieters.

Free 100! foods must have 100 calories or less per serving, such as frozen novelties, 100-calorie snack bars, and 100-calorie snack bags. Salty, sweet, hot or cold . . . it doesn't matter. What does matter is that it is 100 calories or less. Check the labels carefully to be certain of serving size.

A few pointers:

1. If desired, you may save up 100-calorie allotments of your Free 100! to later spend in one sitting. The thing to remember is that 700 calories is 700 calories, whether you eat them in one day or over seven. If you've scheduled a celebratory or splurge meal and want to save up your calories for it, you can do that. Just keep track of how many calories have accumulated.

2. Please keep in mind that a Free 100! should never be a bad boyfriend food, even in a 100-calorie portion-size package. Otherwise, you'll first start to eat that food more often, and before you know it the quantity you eat will be increasing too. If this happens, pick another food for your Free 100!

3. *A special note on alcoholic beverages:* You may have alcohol on the diet, as long as it falls under your Free 100! One light beer, one shot of hard liquor (80 proof), and four ounces of dry white or red wine are all 100-calorie portions. As a rule, I tend to have clients avoid using soda as their Free 100! so as to avoid getting a large portion for their 100 calories, and also because the sugar can stimulate the appetite.

CHAPTER 14

The Skinny Jeans Diet Recipes

CHOSE THESE RECIPES BECAUSE THEY ARE EASY TO MAKE, THEY are nutritious, they use ingredients you probably have in your kitchen right now, and most important, they taste great!

Breakfast

MORNING PEANUT BUTTER CUP SANDWICH

SERVES 1

Satisfy a chocolate craving at breakfast? Absolutely! For this recipe, you don't need to know how to cook—you just have to assemble.

1 deep chocolate Vitalicious Vitamuffin VitaTop
1 tablespoon fat-free whipped topping (such as Cool Whip Free), thawed

1 teaspoon Better'n Peanut Butter

1. Carefully cut the skinny muffin topper in half lengthwise, so that you have two thin muffin tops. Microwave the halves on high for 10 seconds.
2. In a small bowl, combine the whipped topping and peanut butter. Evenly spread over the skinny muffin topper halves and sandwich together.

Nutrition Information:
162 calories, 5 grams fat, 5.5 grams protein, 10.5 grams fiber

SKINNY JEANS DIET ALBA 70 SHAKE

SERVES 1

Sometimes we want to eat our calories, and other times we want to drink them. This recipe uses pudding mix as a thickener and unsweetened almond milk to boost the flavor, making it taste just like your favorite chocolate milkshake, while keeping the calories in check.

1 packet Alba 70 Snack Shake Mix

1 tablespoon Jell-O Instant sugar-free, fat-free, reduced-calorie pudding and pie filling mix, chocolate flavor

1 cup unsweetened chocolate Almond Breeze almond milk

Place all the ingredients in a shaker cup and shake. To make this drink even thicker, add a cup of crushed ice and blend for one minute.

Nutrition Information:
145 calories, 3.6 grams fat, 2.2 grams protein, 1.5 grams fiber

BERRY GOOD SMOOTHIE

SERVES 1

Smoothies are packed with nutrition and taste like dessert. Even your kids will ask for one! Using high-fiber, frozen berries gives this recipe a thick, frozen consistency. If you can't drink it through a straw, grab the closest spoon!

1 cup frozen blueberries	½ cup unsweetened vanilla
½ cup frozen blackberries	Almond Breeze almond
1 tablespoon vanilla extract	milk

Place the frozen berries in the blender and allow them to thaw slightly, about two minutes. Add the vanilla and almond milk. Blend at medium-high speed until smooth.

Nutrition Information:
180 calories, 3 grams fat, 2 grams protein, 8.5 grams fiber

MEXICAN MICROWAVE EGG SCRAMBLE

SERVES 1

Not patient enough to make an omelet? Or maybe you just don't have the time to cook it? Here's your answer—this egg scramble is fast and easy, and there's only one mug and fork to clean up!

Nonstick cooking spray

½ cup liquid egg substitute

2 tablespoons salsa

¼ cup shredded, reduced-fat Mexican cheese

Salt and pepper, to taste

1. Coat a large, microwave-safe coffee mug with nonstick cooking spray. Add the egg substitute and salsa and whisk with a fork until well blended. Microwave on high for 45 seconds.
2. Stir in the cheese and microwave on high for 30 seconds, or until the eggs are set. Add salt and pepper to taste.

Nutrition Information:
150 calories, 6 grams fat, 20 grams protein, 0.5 grams fiber

Lunch

BARBECUE CHICKEN PIZZA

SERVES 2

This pizza features two surprises. The first is BBQ sauce, and the second is the huge portion!

1 100-calorie high-fiber wrap, any brand

½ cup low-fat tomato sauce, such as Ragu Light (60 calories or less per ½-cup serving)

3 ounces diced, boneless, skinless chicken breast, tossed with 2 tablespoons barbecue sauce

1 cup diced onions and peppers

1 ounce reduced-fat, part-skim mozzarella cheese

1. Preheat the oven to 350°F.
2. Spread the tomato sauce over the tortilla. Cover with the chicken and vegetables. Sprinkle with cheese and place in the oven for 5 to 7 minutes.

Nutrition Information:
203 calories, 6 grams fat, 20 grams protein, 6 grams fiber

SKINNY EGG WHITE SALAD

SERVES 1

This yolkless salad is great in the summertime. You can add diced celery and onion to kick up the flavor. This recipe is perfect when cooking for one since it makes a single, huge serving!

5 hard-boiled eggs, whites only, chopped

1 tablespoon chopped fresh chives

2 teaspoons Hellmann's Dijonnaise Mustard-Mayonnaise Blend

1 tablespoon Hellmann's Light Mayonnaise

1 packet zero-calorie sweetener (optional)

15 oriental rice crackers, for serving

1. In a large bowl, combine the egg whites, chives, Dijonnaise, mayonnaise, and sweetener.
2. Spread the egg white mixture evenly over the rice crackers and serve.

Nutrition Information:
240 calories, 3.5 grams fat, 2 grams protein, 0.6 grams fiber

Dinner

POTATO CHIP FISH

SERVES 1

This good-for-you fish dish uses white fish, which is very low in calories. If you don't like fish, feel free to substitute chicken. And we all know that adding potato chips to any dish just makes it more fun!

Nonstick cooking spray
1 5-ounce piece of cod or
    other white fish
1 teaspoon honey mustard

1 ounce Baked! Lays
    Original Potato Chips
    (about 12 chips), crushed
Nonstick olive oil spray

1. Preheat the oven to 350°F.
2. Place the fish on a baking sheet sprayed with nonstick cooking spray. Spread the honey mustard on top of the fish. Bake for 10 minutes.
3. Remove fish from oven. Sprinkle crushed potato chips on top of the fish. Mist the chips lightly with nonstick spray, and return to oven. Bake for another 5 minutes, or until golden brown.

Nutrition Information:
278 calories, 3 grams fat, 34 grams protein, 2 grams fiber

SIMPLE SALMON

SERVES 4

The oil found in fish is known for reducing the risk of heart attacks, lowering blood pressure, and bringing down high triglycerides. Plus, this dish is so quick and easy to make that you won't even know you cooked!

1 pound salmon fillet	1 cup Newman's Own
3 garlic cloves	Low-Fat Sesame Ginger
	Salad Dressing (or other
	light sesame soy dressing
	with 50 calories or less per
	2-tablespoon serving)

1. Pat the salmon dry and use a fork to poke holes in the fillet. Rub the fillet with the garlic cloves.
2. Place the salmon, garlic cloves, and dressing in a resealable bag. Marinate for 30 minutes, or up to 5 hours.
3. Preheat the oven to 350°F.
4. Transfer the salmon to a baking sheet and discard the marinade and garlic. Bake for 12 to 13 minutes, or until cooked to your liking. Remove the salmon from the oven and preheat the broiler.
5. Place the salmon under the broiler for about 4 minutes. The salmon can be served hot or at room temperature. Cut the salmon into 4 pieces and serve.

Nutrition Information:
217 calories, 9.5 grams fat, 29 grams protein, 0.5 grams carbohydrates

QUICK, SKINNY CHILI

SERVES 4

This chili is fresh and light, but makes for a great meal at football parties! Add more vegetables to decrease the calories per bite and increase the volume in your bowl.

Nonstick spray
1 pound extra-lean ground
   turkey or beef (such as
   Laura's Lean Beef)
1 medium onion, chopped
1 garlic clove, minced
4 teaspoons chili powder

½ teaspoon salt
1 8-ounce can tomato sauce
1 14.5-ounce can chopped
   tomatoes with basil, garlic,
   and oregano
1 cup chopped red pepper

1. Spray a large sauté pan with nonstick spray and heat it over medium-high heat. Add the turkey, onion, and garlic and cook until the turkey is browned and cooked through, breaking it up with a wooden spoon.
2. Add the rest of the ingredients, cover, and simmer for 15 minutes.

Nutrition Information:
251 calories, 8.7 grams fat, 25.8 grams protein, 4.7 grams fiber

STEAK STIR-FRY

SERVES 1

A great way to satisfy die-hard meat eaters with a reasonable 5-ounce serving of steak.

5 ounces top round steak, cut in strips

1 crushed garlic clove

3 tablespoons beef broth, fat removed

1 cup chopped Chinese cabbage

1 cup sliced mushrooms

1 cup broccoli florets

½ cup pea pods

1. Sauté the steak and garlic in the broth. When the meat is almost cooked through, add the vegetables.
2. Cover and steam for a few minutes, until the vegetables are tender-crisp. Sprinkle with soy sauce to taste.

Nutrition Information:
300 calories, 8 grams fat, 46 grams protein, 6 grams fiber

CAULIFLOWER "FLATBREAD"

SERVES 2

Flatbreads may be a popular menu item, but the calories they pack can keep us from fitting into our favorite pants. This flatbread uses cauliflower in place of wheat, saving calories without sacrificing taste. Making it at home means you can use part-skim mozzarella (or mix half the cheese with the fat-free variety for even fewer calories). Here is a "lite" version that cooks up in as much time as it takes your waiter to bring your order!

Nonstick spray

1 cup finely shredded part-skim mozzarella cheese

4 cups diced, cooked cauliflower

½ cup liquid egg substitute

1 teaspoon minced garlic

1 teaspoon dried Italian herbs

1. Preheat the oven to 400°F and prepare a square baking pan with nonstick spray. Set aside.
2. In a medium bowl, combine all the ingredients. Use a potato masher or your hands to mash well. Transfer the mixture to the pan and smooth it flat. Bake for 10 minutes, then lower the oven to 350°F and bake for 20 minutes more, or until the "flatbread" is cooked through.
3. Cut the "flatbread" in half to make 2 servings.

Nutrition Information:
250 calories, 11 grams fat, 25 grams protein, 7grams fiber

SKINNY MEATLOAF

SERVES 5

This is a super-simple recipe with very little cleanup. Now that's the way I like it!

MEATLOAF

Nonstick spray

¼ cup ketchup

¼ cup low-sugar apricot, strawberry, or grape jelly

1 pound lean ground turkey or beef (such as Laura's Lean Beef)

½ cup chopped onion

½ cup chopped carrot

¼ cup instant oats

¼ cup liquid egg substitute

¼ teaspoon salt

¼ teaspoon pepper

TOPPING

2 tablespoons ketchup

1 tablespoon low-sugar apricot, strawberry, or grape jelly

1. Preheat the oven to 400°F and prepare a loaf pan with nonstick spray.
2. To make the meatloaf, combine the ketchup, jelly, turkey, onion, carrot, oats, egg substitute, salt, and pepper in a large bowl. Transfer the mixture to the pan and smooth the top with a spoon.

3. To make the topping, mix the ketchup and jelly in a small bowl. Spread evenly over the loaf.

4. Bake the meatloaf for 50 minutes, or until the top is browned and the meatloaf is cooked through.

Nutrition Information:

205 calories, 6.7 grams fat, 20.5 grams protein, 1.2 grams fiber

TOFU "NOODLES" WITH ROASTED VEGETABLES

SERVES 2

You'll never believe that the pasta in this dish is really tofu. It's the biggest and greatest fake-out ever!

Nonstick spray
2 cups sliced zucchini
2 cups peeled, sliced carrots
2 cups sliced eggplant
Kosher salt

2 bags Nasoya Pasta Zero Plus
   Shiratake Tofu Noodles
   (linguine or spaghetti style)
1 tablespoon Best Life Butter
   Spread (or other butter
   spread with 50 calories per
   tablespoon)

1. Preheat the oven to 425°F. Prepare a baking sheet with nonstick spray.
2. Spread all the vegetables in a single layer on the baking sheet. Spray the vegetables with nonstick spray and sprinkle with salt. Roast for 15 minutes, or until the vegetables are cooked through.
3. Meanwhile, cook the tofu noodles according to the package directions. Strain and pat dry with paper towels to absorb all the moisture. (This step is very important if you don't want watery tofu noodles. Dry very well!) Place the noodles in a serving bowl and gently mix in the butter spread.
4. Toss in the roasted vegetables and serve.

Nutrition Information:
203 calories, 5.5 grams fat, 7 grams protein, 8 grams fiber

THAT'S A CROCK OF VEGGIES

SERVES 4

A slow cooker is a must for a busy family. This recipe takes five minutes to put together. You can even do it the night before and refrigerate it overnight.

3 cups cubed butternut
squash
3 cups peeled, sliced carrots
3 cups cubed eggplant

½ cup chopped onion
1 15-ounce can vegetable
broth (or 2 cups packaged
broth)

1. Combine the squash, carrots, eggplant, and onion in a slow cooker. Pour the broth on top. Cover and cook on high for 4 to 5 hours, or until the vegetables are tender (exact timing is not critical with slow cooking).
2. Mix well before serving.

Nutritional Information:
130 calories, 0.5 grams fat, 3 grams protein, 9 grams fiber

LEMON CHICKEN THIGHS WITH OLIVES AND CAPERS

SERVES 4

Having company and don't want to spend all day in the kitchen? This dish is so good and pretty that you can serve it proudly, and you won't break a sweat. Or make it for your family and they'll feel like honored guests!

Nonstick cooking spray
¼ cup flour
¼ teaspoon salt
¼ teaspoon ground black pepper
8 boneless, skinless chicken thighs

1 cup packaged chicken broth
2 tablespoons lemon juice
2 tablespoons capers
2 tablespoons chopped black olives

1. Coat a 12-inch nonstick skillet with cooking spray and set it over medium-high heat.
2. In a small bowl, combine the flour, salt, and black pepper. Rub or sprinkle the flour mixture all over the chicken to coat it.
3. Add the chicken to the skillet in a single layer and cook until browned, about 5 minutes. Turn the chicken over and cook until golden brown and cooked through, about 4 minutes more. Remove the chicken from the skillet and set aside.

4. Pour the broth into the skillet and scrape any browned chicken bits remaining from the bottom of the pan and discard. Return the chicken to the skillet, cover, and reduce heat to low. The broth will reduce. Simmer until heated through, about 3 minutes.

5. Stir in the lemon juice, capers, and olives, and cook about 1 minute.

6. Place 2 chicken thighs on each plate. Top with the capers and olives and drizzle with the remaining sauce and serve.

Nutrition Information:

200 calories, 6 grams fat, 28 grams protein, 0.6 grams fiber

CLAM ME UP SPAGHETTI SQUASH

SERVES 4

The traditional dish of spaghetti with white clam sauce can clock in at 480 calories per cup. Ouch! Here's a great good guy alternative with a secret ingredient (shh ... spaghetti squash)!

1 medium spaghetti squash

1 6.5-ounce can baby clams
  or 6 ounces fresh clams

Nonstick cooking spray

1 teaspoon olive oil

1 medium onion, diced

2 garlic cloves, minced

10 cherry tomatoes, halved

2 tablespoons chopped
  parsley

1¼ cups chicken broth

1 tablespoon cornstarch

1. Soften the spaghetti squash by cooking it in the microwave for about 2 minutes on high. Cut the squash in half lengthwise and scrape out the seeds. Microwave for 10 more minutes. Alternatively, bake the squash at 400°F until softened, about 40 minutes.

2. Remove the flesh of the squash by shredding it with a fork into a large colander. Set it aside to drain.

3. Drain the clams. Spray a large nonstick skillet with cooking spray. Heat the oil over medium-high heat, add the onion, and cook until soft, about 5 minutes. Stir in the garlic and cook 30 seconds more. Add the tomatoes, stir, and cook for 1 minute. Reduce the heat to low and stir in the clams and parsley.

4. Bring the chicken broth to a boil in a small pan over medium heat. Combine the cornstarch and 1 tablespoon water in a small bowl. Whisk the cornstarch slurry into the boiling broth and cook for 1 minute to thicken.

5. Pat the squash dry with paper towels or a cloth napkin. Do this really well so your dish isn't watery! Mix the squash into the clam sauce, toss, and serve.

Nutrition Information:
170 calories, 3 grams fat, 14 grams protein, 4.5 grams fiber

EASIEST SPAGHETTI SQUASH EVER!

SERVES 3 (MAKES 2–2 1/2 CUPS)

You can load the crockpot in less than a minute with this recipe! Make sure you get a spaghetti squash that will fit whole into your slow cooker. A small to medium squash is perfect for an average 2-quart cooker.

1 small to medium spaghetti squash

(optional for serving) Butter spray, a sprinkle of grated Parmesan, your favorite light tomato sauce (any tomato sauce with 50 to 60 calories per standard ½-cup serving size)

1. Pierce the spaghetti squash with a fork in several places. Add it to the slow cooker with ½ cup of water and cook on low for 6 to 7 hours.
2. Cut the squash lengthwise, scoop out the seeds, and scrape the flesh into a large bowl with a fork. Pat dry with paper towels or a cloth napkin.
3. Serve with your favorite toppings.

Nutritional Information:
105 calories, 1 gram fat, 3 grams protein, 5.4 grams fiber

EASY PLEASING SLOW COOKER BEEF STEW

SERVES 5

Dense vegetables, such as carrots, can take as long to cook as some cuts of meat. When adding the ingredients to a slow cooker, make sure you place the root vegetables on the bottom of the pot; then add the lean protein, seasonings, other vegetables, and liquid. This keeps the vegetables moist during cooking.

4 cups baby carrots

1 medium onion, thickly
   chopped

1/3 cup flour

Salt and pepper, to taste

1 pound beef stew meat

1 14-ounce can diced
   tomatoes, undrained

1. Place the carrots and onion in the bottom of a slow cooker.
2. In a small bowl, mix the flour, salt, and pepper and toss with the beef to coat. Add to the slow cooker with the tomatoes and 2 cups water.
3. Cover the slow cooker and cook on low for 7 to 8 hours, or until the beef and carrots are tender.

Nutritional Information:
218 calories, 4 grams fat, 23.5 grams protein, 4.2 grams fiber

EASIEST ROASTED VEGETABLES EVER!

SERVES 5

If you think vegetables are boring without butter and cream sauce, think again. Here's a fast and simple way to make delicious roasted vegetables. Remember, veggies should take up the most real estate on your plate!

Nonstick spray
2 cups sliced zucchini (or
   your favorite veggie)

2 cups sliced red or yellow
   bell peppers
1 cup sliced eggplant
Kosher salt

1. Preheat the oven to 425°F. Spray a large baking sheet with nonstick spray.
2. Spread the vegetables in a single layer on the baking sheet. Spray the vegetables with nonstick spray and sprinkle with salt. Roast for 15 minutes, or until the vegetables are cooked through.

Nutritional Information:
26 calories, 0.3 grams fat, 1 gram protein, 2 grams fiber

Sides

MOCK MASHED POTATOES

SERVES 4

Cauliflower has great cancer-fighting antioxidants, making this dish extra healthy! On top of that, these "mashed potatoes" are so creamy that your family will never know they aren't the real deal.

2 16-ounce bags frozen
cauliflower florets
1 small Russet potato,
unpeeled and cut into
rough cubes
¼ cup skim milk

1 tablespoon butter spread,
such as Brummel and
Brown
½ teaspoon salt
garlic to taste

1. Bring a large pot of water to a boil over high heat.
2. Add the cauliflower and potato to the pot and return to a boil. Reduce the heat to medium and cook for 20 minutes, or until the cauliflower and potatoes are fork-tender.
3. Drain the water and return the potato and cauliflower to the pot. Mash with potato masher until roughly smooth.
4. Add the milk, butter, salt, and garlic. Mash again until completely smooth.

Nutritional Information:
81 calories, 0.6 grams fat, 5 grams protein, 7 grams fiber

SKINNY JEANS SPINACH SOUFFLÉ

SERVES 6

Popeye won't be the only one who loves to eat his spinach. Not only is this soufflé full of protein, fiber, and vitamins, but one cup of raw spinach has just 7 calories!

1½ cups fat-free ricotta cheese

1½ cups part-skim ricotta cheese

3 10-ounce packages frozen spinach, thawed and drained

4 egg whites

½ cup whole-wheat flour

3 tablespoons grated Parmesan cheese

1 tablespoon ground nutmeg

1 tablespoon garlic powder

Dash of salt and pepper

1. Preheat the oven to 350°F.
2. Combine all the ingredients in a large bowl.
3. Spread the mixture evenly in an 8-inch-square baking dish. Bake for 30 minutes, or until slightly browned on top.

Nutrition Information:
220 calories, 6.6 grams fat, 18 grams protein, 5 grams fiber

GREEN BEANS

SERVES 4

If green bean casserole is one of your holiday favorites, this will be a close second. It's also a great way to add a little festivity to any weeknight meal.

Nonstick spray
1 10¾-ounce can 98 percent fat-free cream of mushroom soup, condensed

2 14.5-ounce cans French-style green beans, drained (or 4 cups trimmed fresh green beans)
Garlic powder, to taste
Salt and pepper, to taste
¼ cup panko bread crumbs

1. Preheat the oven to 350°F. Spray an 8-inch-square baking dish with nonstick spray.
2. Add the soup, green beans, garlic, and salt and pepper to the baking dish, and mix to combine.
3. Smooth out the mixture and sprinkle the top evenly with bread crumbs. Bake for 25 minutes, or until golden on top.

Nutritional Information:
123 calories, 2.6 grams fat, 3.5 grams protein, 1 gram fiber

CRAZY GLAZY CARROTS

SERVES 4 (1-CUP SERVINGS)

Slow-cooking makes for a nice, stress-free meal—and it makes the house smell really good too! In addition, cleanup is a breeze. Buy a slow cooker with a removable inside crock and you'll go from cooktop to tabletop all in one appliance.

1 16-ounce package baby carrots
¼ cup sugar-free apricot jelly
1 tablespoon Splenda Brown Sugar Blend
½ teaspoon light butter spread (such as Brummel and Brown)

¼ teaspoon ground nutmeg
½ teaspoon ground cinnamon
1 tablespoon cornstarch
2 tablespoons cold water

1. Combine all the ingredients except the cornstarch in a slow cooker. Cook on low for 7 hours.
2. Before serving, make a paste of the cornstarch and water and stir it into the carrots. Cook for 15 minutes, or until nicely thickened, and serve.

Nutritional Information:
110 calories, 0.7 grams fat, 1.4 grams protein, 3 grams fiber

SPEEDY, SKINNY POTATO FRIES

SERVES 1

These are a favorite with kids and grown-ups alike—fast to make, inexpensive, and filling. Plus, there's only one plate to clean up!

Nonstick olive oil cooking spray
1 medium Russet potato, unpeeled, cut into thin lengthwise spears

Dash of salt
Dash of paprika

1. Spray a microwavable plate with nonstick cooking spray. Spread the potato spears in a single layer on the plate and lightly spray again. Sprinkle with salt and paprika.
2. Microwave for about 8 minutes (or whatever the baked potato setting on your microwave indicates), until the spears are crisp like thick-cut French fries.

Nutritional Information:
131 calories, 0.3 grams fat, 4 grams protein, 3.5 grams fiber

Desserts

SKINNY JEANS BAKED APPLE

SERVES 1

This is the perfect way to get the taste of apple pie for less than 100 calories per serving! Who says a satisfying dessert has to be high in calories?

1 medium apple, any variety, unpeeled, cored and cut into cubes

1 packet zero-calorie sweetener

½ teaspoon apple pie spice (or ground cinnamon)

Place the apple cubes in a microwave-safe bowl and sprinkle with the sweetener and spice. Microwave for 3 minutes, until softened.

Nutrition Information:
85 calories, 0.3 grams fat, 0.3 grams protein, 4.5 grams fiber

SKINNY S'MORES

SERVES 1

Ninety-five percent of dieters fall off their diets because they feel deprived. Try this amazing take on s'mores and say hello to dessert and good-bye to deprivation for good!

1 graham cracker (2 squares)	6 milk chocolate chips
1 large marshmallow	

1. Break the graham cracker into two squares. Tear the marshmallow in half and place one marshmallow half on each square. Press 3 chocolate chips into each marshmallow.
2. Put in the toaster oven, open-faced, for one toast cycle, or until the marshmallow is golden and the chocolate is melted. Press the graham cracker halves together to make one s'more.

Nutritional Information:
100 calories, 2.6 grams fat, 1 gram protein, 0.6 grams fiber

SKINNY BAKED PEARS

SERVES 4

This recipe hits the mark on both great flavor and great nutrition. It makes a delicious dessert, but don't feel guilty eating it for breakfast too!

Nonstick cooking spray
4 medium pears, halved,
    cored, and peeled

¼ cup Splenda Brown Sugar
    Blend
½ teaspoon ground
    cinnamon

1. Preheat the oven to 350°F. Spray a baking sheet with nonstick cooking spray.
2. Toss the pears in a bowl with the sweetener and cinnamon, coating well.
3. Place the pears core side up and 2 inches apart on the baking sheet. (Alternatively, use a muffin pan sprayed with nonstick spray and stand the pears upright.) Bake for 30 minutes, or until the pears are softened.

Nutritional Information:
144 calories, 0.6 grams fat, 0.6 grams protein, 3.5 grams fiber

Acknowledgments

THIS BOOK NEVER WOULD HAVE SEEN THE LIGHT OF DAY IF IT weren't for Shelby Meizlik, who saw potential in the work I was doing, believed in me personally, and brought this book to the right people at HarperCollins.

I also must thank the talented health journalist David Nayor, whose editorial guidance, organization, integrity, passion, and unending patience helped me along the way. He is simply the best. I also want to thank veteran food writer Jean Tang, who helped give this book some sass and its no-nonsense girl voice. Thank you both for keeping me calm, sane, and focused.

I am especially grateful to Cassie Jones, my super-talented and dedicated editor at HarperCollins. Cassie guided me through my first writing experience and was instrumental in taking *The Skinny Jeans Diet* from concept to reality.

Right beside me throughout this process were the people who inspire me every day—my clients. Without them, there would be no Skinny Jeans Diet. They are my greatest teachers, and because of them I love my work.

And last on this list, but first in my life, my most heartfelt gratitude goes to my family. To my mom and dad, who have believed in me and loved me unconditionally for a lifetime. I am so grateful, and love and thank you.

To my husband, Stephen, who sees the best and overlooks the worst in me. I couldn't ask for anything better than loving and being loved by you. And to Alix and Evan, who are the reason I live. Being your mother is truly the pleasure of my life. I am one helluva lucky girl.

Index